Intermittent Fa
#1 Complete B
Guide to Lose Weight Fast

By Robert McGowan BSc.

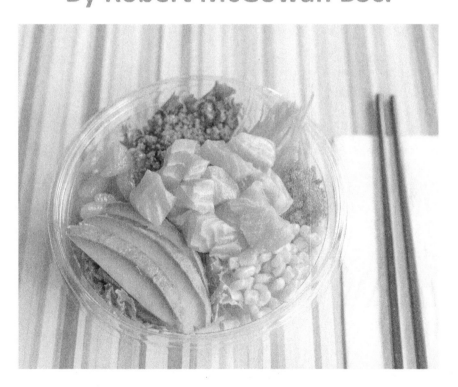

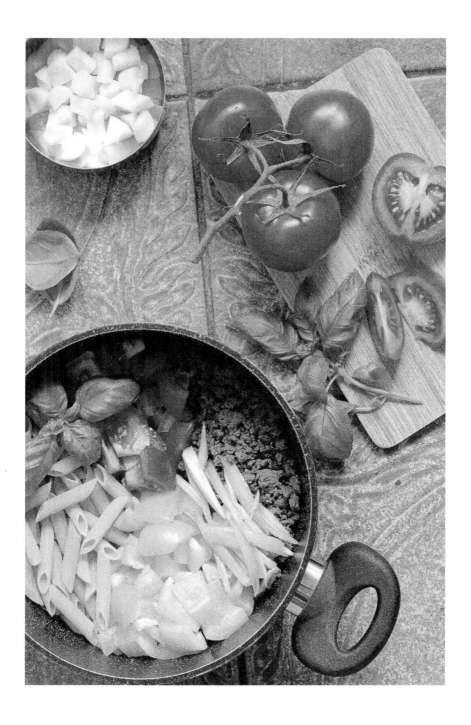

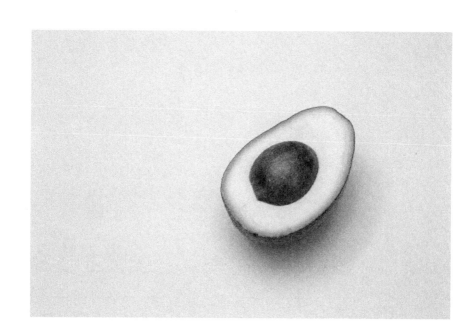

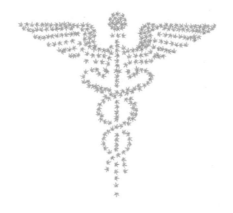

Contents

Preface

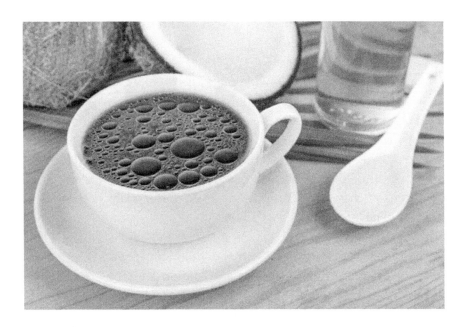

Psst! Yes you!

So, you want to know the secret of getting into the **best shape of your life**, without having to go on a diet?

Well then let's begin!

But first I'd like to say a big warm, 'thank you' for buying this book, and I want to congratulate you for taking the first major step towards a leaner, healthier and fitter you.

I love sharing what I've learned, and I am genuinely thrilled to have the opportunity to share my knowledge and personal experience with you. I get so much from knowing that I've helped people make the transition from being overweight and unhappy into a thinner, happier, energetic version of themselves. It's like a completely different person emerges.

With this book I have condensed everything that I've learned through trial and error over the years and created a piece of work with one major goal in mind.

To help **YOU** achieve rapid weight loss and to guide you towards looking and feeling amazing.

Now, the number 1 reason why most people fail to lose any weight is because they fail to take massive action. It's as simple as that. That's why, before we go much further I would very much love for you to consider making the conscious decision right now to follow and action the step by step guidance set out in this book so that you too can get the same mind-blowing results which I and others have done.

You have got the power to do this. The instructions are all right here waiting for you.

All you've got to do now is read it, digest it and most importantly to take-action. If you are willing to do this then the incredible results will soon speak for themselves.

Right, with that said we'll get straight to it shall we?

I'd like you to consider this for a moment.

When you hear the words 'Intermittent Fasting' what's the first thing that you think of?

- Starving yourself and feeling miserable?

- Doing without the food you love and constantly counting calories? (and feeling quite miserable)
- Or perhaps it's enduring a hellish period of only eating bland food or boring, tasteless meal replacement bars? Not getting the results you want (and yes, you've guessed it, feeling rather miserable!)

I must admit that when I first heard the term, 'Intermittent Fasting' being used it didn't exactly ignite a fire in me to want to give it a go. I love my food and drink too much and fasting sounds like having to starve yourself. Hmm starving myself is not, and never will be on my radar for things to try. Life's too short for that.

Delving a bit deeper however piqued my interest enough to begin some initial research. It didn't take long before the topic became very interesting to me albeit the sensational health benefit claims initially seemed a bit too good to be true especially since no reduction in calories or any exercise was required to get real life changing results.

Now this was something that I could do!

Here was a simple method of eating-not dieting-which claimed to have dramatic positive effects on your physical and mental health AND programed your body to burn stubborn fat fast!

You would not be required to deny yourself the food that you love, and you will not go hungry. You will no longer find yourself staring off into space in the grocery isle as you mentally tally the calories/carbs/protein/fat content on food labels while trying to work out if it fits in with your current calorific daily requirements.

No more following pointless 'point' systems or running like Usain Bolt on the treadmill while your chiseled and beady eyed personal trainer glares at you!

More importantly you will not be trying and failing with another fad diet that's just unsustainable, long term.

You too might be thinking at this point that this all sounds a bit too good to be true however make no mistake, the secret methods which you are about to discover will quickly produce very dramatic effects.

Practically anyone who wants to get lean can do this, no matter what your age or current fitness levels. More importantly, YOU can do this. And I'll show you exactly how to do it safely and effectively.

This method of eating will particularly suit you if:

You want to lose weight fast and keep it off long term.

You have tried dieting and it didn't work.

You want to look and feel amazing.

You're too busy to exercise.

A little bit about me. I am a practicing herbalist, nutritionist, personal trainer and chef. I have a real passion for eating well and I've spent my entire life studying food, nutrition, exercise, and sports psychology. I have successfully utilized various diets and health supplements and I am passionate about health, fitness and mental wellbeing. I have trained in the martial arts including Bruce Lees JKD and Kick Boxing, and I enjoy weight training, running, rock climbing and cycling. That's not to say that I'm an extremist. I am most certainly not. I do love feeling fit and full of energy however I am a firm believer in living one's life to the full and if that means enjoying your favorite foods and wine or whatever on occasion then that's absolutely fine by me. It's all about balance after all and living the life you love. What's the point being lean but unhappy and feeling that you're denying yourself of life's pleasures?

When it comes to exercise and nutrition, my curious, inquisitive and at times unconventional nature has often led me to push the boundaries to get to the truth on what really works and what doesn't. You are probably aware of the fact that the health and fitness industry can be full of mis information, usually with the aim of trying to sell you something that probably don't need at all. I never just take what I read as gospel truth. I always experiment, test and tweak things until I find a solution that I know works 100%. I have used this knowledge to help hundreds of clients successfully lose weight and get in the best shape of their live. It's really not that difficult once you know what to do and implement it.

My goal with this book was too take all that I have learned and create the best, most valuable one stop 'IF' resource available to help you get on the best shape of your life. This book is designed to be easy to understand and most importantly, to get you the results that you want in the quickest time frame possible.

It is my true belief that every single reader of this book who takes-action will be amazed at how different they look and feel and that this change will have a positive knock on effect on all other areas of their lives.

When you successfully set then achieve your fitness goals your confidence will go through the roof. This positivity and new-found energy will impact upon your relationships and your family life, your productivity, your working life, your business and your ability to set and achieve even more goals.

Can you imagine yourself in your new clothes looking leaner, fitter and full of vitality? How good will it feel to finally look in the mirror and love what you see in front of you? It's exciting and powerful stuff and I can't wait to show you how to do it!

Thanks once again for buying this book. I really do hope that you love it. If you do feel that you have gained real value from it then please take two minutes to leave me an honest review view by clicking here http://www.Amazon.com/gp/customer-reviews/write-a-review.html?asin=B07NQQY5TZ

It's quick and easy and it will help others decide if they too could benefit from the book. Thanks in advance.

Are you ready? I'm ready!

Now let's get started!

Introduction

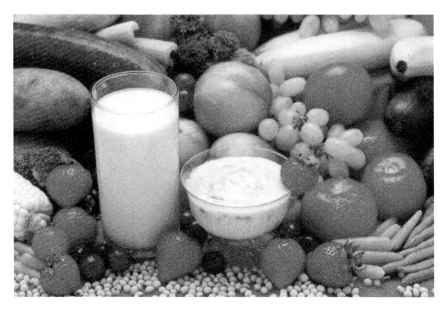

There are many diets out there designed to help you lose weight. I have tried and tested most of them. You will hear about the Atkins Diet, the South Beach Diet, and Weight Watchers. Worse yet, you may resort to doing the more extreme crash diets such as the Cabbage Soup Diet or the Military Diet. But, while these extreme fad and crash diets may have quite a few people purporting their benefits, they can actually be harmful to you. These diets will help you lose weight quickly. Yet, in the long term, they will damage your metabolism and cause you to gain more weight than you had originally lost.

You don't have to resort to these harmful diets in order to lose weight. Instead, you can use intermittent fasting to lose weight while promoting your health and metabolism. Rather than starving yourself, you can enjoy short fasts broken up with periods of eating all the delicious calories your body needs.

Many may worry that intermittent fasting is similar to the juice and other cleanses, which deprive your body of many calories it requires. With these cleanses you are deficient in nutrients and can become weak and hungry. Although, there is no need to fear. Intermittent fasting not only has a centuries-long successful history but, many studies have also proven its benefits to both weight loss and health. Put simply you are able to enjoy the same number of calories and foods you usually eat, and still lose weight.

Within the pages of this book, you will find all the information you need to begin intermittent fasting, whether you are a complete beginner or have moderate experience with fasting. This book doesn't provide dubious claims. Instead, you will find scientifically backed data in an easy to read format. Why wait to begin a journey toward better weight and manageable weight loss? With the tools provided within this book, you can succeed and reach your weight loss goals.

Chapter 1:

Intermittent Fasting Defined

What is Intermittent Fasting?

Unlike when people go long periods without eating and depriving their body of nutrients, intermittent fasting is based on going moderate amount of time periods without eating. You are still consuming all the nutrients your body requires, but this allows you to lose weight more easily. Believe it or not, there are even many proven significant health benefits. It's basically a pattern of skipping meals, and it's something that is used on a regular basis by many people. In fact, it has a rooted history in ancient medicine and many world religions. The major world religions of Christianity, Islam, and Judaism all have some form of fasting periods in their religious calendars.

We have even found evidence of fasting having been used medicinally and therapeutically within the Ancient Grecian culture. Many physicians, including the famed Hippocrates, would prescribe intermittent fasting for their patients. This was especially promoted for people with low appetites.

Traditionally within the Jewish religion people will fast for six days out of the year. Although, fasting is not allowed during Sabbath, except for Yom Kippur. During the time of Yom Kippur, every man and woman (those above the age of bat mitzvah and bar mitzvah) are expected to fast unless it would dangerously affect their health. During this fast, the people refrain from all food and drink, which includes water.

While not all Christians fast, there are many Christian denominations which practice fasting from time to time. Sometimes this will be for specific times and seasons, but it is also commonly practiced when they feel led by the Holy Spirit to fast for a specific reason. For instance, someone may fast when they are searching for an answer to a problem or praying for healing. For Western, Christianity fasting is most often practiced by Catholics, Methodists, Anglicans, and Reformed Baptists. This is most prominent during the time of Lent, which is a partial fast that lasts forty days in order to represent Christ's time within the desert.

The way in which people choose to fast within Christianity varies greatly not only depending on the denomination but from person to person. Some people may choose to practice intermittent fasting on a daily basis. Whereas other people may only fast on Good Friday and Ash Wednesday.

Within Buddhism, monks and nuns will often intermittent fast after lunch each day. They have found that this is not only food for discipline and meditation, but also increased health.
Within the Hindu religion, similarly, as within the Christian religion, there is no one set standard of fasting. Depending on a person's local customs and individual beliefs the way they practice intermittent fasting can greatly differ. Sometimes people

will only eat a single meal during the day, some refrain from eating specific types of food, and others may fast between the hours of sunset and sunrise. Many Hindus also have specific holidays and set times for fasting. For instance, they may fast on Tuesdays, during Purim, Ekadashi, Pradosha, or during festivals. Within the Muslim culture, fasting is an extremely important and vital part of their religion. It's seen as not only fasting from food and drink, but also from behaviors that are believed to be immoral. This is especially practiced during the sacred time of Ramadan. Muslims seek to cleanse their body and soul, increasing their good deeds and consciousness. During Ramadan, they will abstain from food and drink during the day and then feast in the evenings.

Along with religious and health-centered fasting, hunger strikes have been used across the globe for centuries in order to make a point to those in power. Some of these hunger strikes, such as those completed by the suffragettes and during India's revolution, have become legendary.

As you can see, restricted eating can mean many things. Intermittent fasting can either mean zero calories or just a very small quantity of food to minimize your caloric intake. The method and plan of intermittent fasting you follow are up to you and the results you want. Some critics will try to equate intermittent fasting with starvation and consider it an extreme and dangerous length to go to. They'll say you're harming your body. Yet, fasting is very different than starvation, and studies have proven this. Starvation means that there's no ending point when a person has nothing to eat. Their nutrition is restricted, causing them to become deficient in many vital nutrients.

Although, when you are fasting, you have the strength to voluntarily choose to give up food for a duration of time. Whether that time will simply be 4 hours or 14 hours, it's up to you, and it's at your discretion as you make that decision based on your bodily needs. Not only that but when you do eat you can ensure that you are eating all that your body requires so that you never become deficient in nutrients.

A lot of people find that intermittent fasting is an extremely effective weight loss plan. How does that work? What fasting does is have the body "turn itself on" to use up the fat already stored as a reserve. When you have no food coming in as a source of fuel, the body recognizes the shortage and forces itself to use what it has stored away for emergencies. That means you're losing that extra fat you can't get rid of. Science proves that when you eat, especially when you have excess carbohydrates in particular, the body stores them as fat molecules or sugar molecules. The process is called De-Novo Lipogenesis which literally means "making fat from new."

The body is an adaptive machine, so when you skip a meal and force it to search for an alternative fuel source, it uses the fat molecules it has stored away. You already had those molecules all along. It's now time to use them for energy.

If other diet plans or adjusting your diet isn't working, sometimes a new and scientifically-backed approach is needed. Whether you choose to skip meals or restrict your eating window in order to have your body remain calorie deficit to encourage weight loss, you may be worried about hunger pangs that can be hard to ignore that you might constantly be watching the clock to see when you can eat again. Yet, while people may show these signs of hunger when they first begin intermittent fasting, over time, your body will adjust, and the process will become easier. You can trust in the fact that research has shown that intermittent fasting has many positive physical and mental health benefits, not just weight loss.

As with any new diet or exercise plan, you will soon adjust fasting to your busy schedule, and it will become easier to handle and incorporate into your day. It makes your life a lot easier when it comes to meals as it allows you to focus on when you can eat instead of what you can eat. You just have to make sure you don't overcompensate by binge eating between fasts. And, that you're eating meals that give you enough energy. You want to be sure you're eating a variety of nutrients from protein, good fats and carbohydrates to give yourself all the vitamins and minerals you need.

Though you can't have any food when fasting, you are encouraged to have non-caloric beverages to stay hydrated. Caffeine is encouraged because it's a substance that reduces the body's hunger pangs and will trick your stomach into feeling fuller than it really is. So, an extra-large cup of coffee without milk or sugar (you can use sweetener) in the morning can make you feel fuller to help to get through your morning fast until it's time for you to break your fasting period.

Intermittent fasting for weight loss may not right for every single person, but it does come with an exciting variety of proven health benefits which will be explored in detail later in this book. It is important to note that if you've ever suffered from an eating disorder, then it is highly recommended that you don't use intermittent fasting as a weight loss tool. Before you decide if intermittent fasting is right for you, you need to consult with your doctor. If you are on any prescription medication that you are required to take on a regular basis, then fasting may not work for you at this time. Many prescription medications need to be taken with food, which will break your fast and keep you from reaping the benefits of this meal plan. If you are fighting obesity and other symptoms like high blood pressure, a doctor might actually recommend a fasting schedule to help you see beneficial health results.

If you wish to commit to intermittent fasting, you should view it as a lifestyle change. If you view it with a casual attitude, then it likely won't work out for you and you will not get the results you want. Your social life will also be a factor. You need to plan ahead if you are going out eating or drinking with friends and family in advance so that it doesn't interfere with your fasting schedule. If you start to obsess over food the moment you start to feel hunger pangs, then this diet may make you miserable. Although, you may also find that with intermittent fasting you can break your obsession with food and create a healthier view of nutrition.

For most people, there is some form of intermittent fasting that will fit their lifestyle and their needs just fine, even if it's just forcing yourself to have an early dinner and late breakfast. Most of the time, you're fasting without even knowing it! Think of it this way, let's say you have dinner by seven in the evening and don't eat any snacks before bedtime. Then, the next morning, you have a cup of coffee but don't manage to eat breakfast until almost eight. That's a twelve hour fast without even knowing it. All intermittent fasting does is urge you to push that window of fasting more routinely so you can gain more health benefits. For example, if you kept drinking just coffee and water for a few more hours and had a late breakfast or early lunch around eleven, then that's a sixteen-hour fasting window you've just completed.

As with any other diet plan or change in lifestyle, it's important you first have all the information you need regarding how intermittent fasting works, what you should eat when you aren't fasting, fasting models, and the health benefits you'll be gaining.

We've mentioned that intermittent fasting comes with scientifically-backed health benefits, but let's go over some of the details. You don't have to take my word for it; there are many studies that all of this knowledge has been gleaned from. Whether you choose to follow a shorter fasting schedule, such as the twelve hours fast, or a longer fasting schedule, you can reap many benefits. Although, most benefits will be seen with a longer fasting schedule for most people, such as the sixteen hours fast. You've most likely heard of the ketogenic diet and all of its amazing benefits. But, did you know that the Ketogenic Diet and intermittent fasting both cause the body to respond in similar ways? Another very interesting and upcoming variation of Keto is the Vegetarian Keto Diet which I've tried and tested recently. The Vegetarian Keto Diet offers up an incredible range of benefits, however many are confused about what it is and how to get started. It for this reason that I've added some bonus material on Vegetarian Keto for you to get started if you're interested.

We know that fasting for set periods of time can help many people lose not only weight but also increase their health.

Whether you do intermittent fasting on its own or pair it with something else like the ketogenic diet, your body is sure to thank you. Now let's look at the health benefits in a bit more detail, shall we? A few of the many health benefits you may experience will include:

Weight Loss-The main goal.

Usually, our bodies are constantly working to digest and burn the calories we have most recently eaten. This means that the excess calories we have eaten in the past build up and slowly increase into body fat. It's hard to get rid of this because most Americans eat every several hours. Never giving their bodies a chance to burn what they have already eaten. Intermittent fasting provides us with an opportunity to burn this fat that is building up rather than ignoring it and allowing it to grow. You can directly combat the source of your weight gain. In fact, a large portion of weight loss attained with intermittent fasting is direct because of the ability it gives your body to burn this excessive fuel source. In a study published in 2014, it was found that when fasting participants experienced a significant amount of weight loss. The study ran for three to twenty-four weeks and depending on how long each participant was on the study they could lose between three and eight percent of total body weight.[12]

The amount of weight you can lose and how quickly you can lose it will vary from person to person. This is because we all have different metabolisms, health and other features that affect weight loss. For instance, one person may have already been

---

[1]https://nutritionj.biomedcentral.com/articles/10.1186/1475-2891-11-98
[2]https://onlinelibrary.wiley.com/doi/full/10.1111/j.1467-789X.2011.00873.x

practicing short intermittent fasts and a healthy diet unknowingly, whereas another person may have been on a diet of cheeseburgers three times a day.

However, you can expect to lose ten to **twenty pounds the first two weeks** that you begin intermittent fasting. After this period, you may continue to lose between two to four pounds a week. Within a month you can go down two pant or dress sizes! If you stick with intermittent fasting, before you know it you can be down twenty, fifty, or even one-hundred pounds. Sound good?

Boosts Metabolism

Crash and fad diets are known to damage metabolism long-term. But, so too can restrictive eating and fasting that lasts longer than thirty-six hours. This is especially apparent as we age when our metabolism already naturally declines. The good news is that intermittent fasting when followed by regular eating habits, not only causes no damage to the metabolism but actually boosts it By practicing regular intermittent fasting, you are able to increase your metabolism, allowing you to burn more body fat all while retaining the important lean muscle mass that our bodies require in order to function.[3]

Increased Growth Hormone-my personal favorite health benefit.

This was one of the main benefits that really interested me. Many people think little of their hormones unless a doctor has

---

[3]https://www.annualreviews.org/doi/abs/10.1146/annurev-nutr-071816-064634

specifically told them that they have a hormone disorder. But our hormones are incredibly important. One of these hormones, most commonly known as the human growth hormone, is vital for our weight. This hormone is produced within our pituitary gland and is responsible for maintaining bone density, brain health, the health of our tissues, increasing muscle mass, and promoting the regeneration and growth of cells.

When you are undergoing a fast, this hormone will naturally increase to high levels within your body. Studies have found that it can raise up to five times its normal level While your hormones need to remain balanced, it is both safe and ideal to increase the human growth hormone. This is because this hormone, sometimes shortened to HGH, often reduces as we age, predisposing us to increased body fat, decreased muscle, and more delicate and thinner skin. Yet, when we increase this hormone studies have found that we can experience greater fat loss, increased muscle strength, stronger bones, and strengthened cardiovascular health.[4]

Converts White Fat into Brown Fat

One amazing aspect of intermittent fasting is that it not only helps you lose fat, but it converts your unhealthy white fat into a much healthier (and important) brown fat Many people are unaware that there are multiple types of fats within our bodies. But, while white fat is known to contribute to disease and aging, brown fat protects our organs and helps our bodies to burn off the white fat. This, of course, leads to weight loss, but also to increased health.[5]

[4]https://www.sciencedirect.com/science/article/pii/S0939475312002578
[5]https://www.sciencedirect.com/science/article/pii/S1550413117305041

Reduced Muscle Loss

I used to think that if I reduced my overall calories then I'd just lose bodyfat. Nope. That's wrong. Yes, I lost some bodyfat but I lost hard earned muscle mass too. Yikes!

People often get excited about weight loss when they begin a crash or fad diet. But what most don't realize is that this weight loss is mostly water weight which will only return and all-important muscle loss. Not only are our muscles important for our strength and energy levels, but our heart is even a muscle Thankfully, a study published in 2011 found that while both intermittent fasting and calorie restriction lead to comparable fat loss, intermittent fasting lead to much less muscle loss than the calorie restriction did.[6]

Increases Energy Levels

The human body is full of cells. Some of these cells are known as mitochondrial cells, which can produce energy from multiple sources. These sources of fuel include protein, fat, carbohydrates, and ketones. While some cells may only be able to utilize one or two of these fuels as an energy source, mitochondrial cells are able to utilize all of these fuels.

This is especially wonderful news for people who are on a low-carb diet because the brain and a few other cells require glucose from carbohydrates in order to be fueled. However, when you are fasting or in a state of ketosis, your body will naturally produce an

---

[6]https://onlinelibrary.wiley.com/doi/full/10.1111/j.1467-789X.2011.00873.x

increased number of mitochondrial cells, helping you to use other fuel sources for energy within the brain.

While the mitochondrial cells may not replace all of your cells that require glucose for fuel, you can still stay satisfied and healthy when fasting or on a ketogenic diet. This is because of the process of gluconeogenesis. This process converts amino acids from the proteins we eat into the small amount of glucose these non-mitochondrial cells require. Between the increase in mitochondrial cells and a healthy amount of fat and protein between fasting periods, you will find your body is well-fueled despite going longer periods without eating.

The process of increased mitochondrial cells naturally increases our energy levels, as well. This is because these cells convert ninety percent of the fuel our bodies require into energy. You will find over time that both your physical and mental energy will increase enough for you to notice it. Many of us need this boost with the on-the-go lifestyle that is common in the Western world and the fatigue often caused by our modern diets.[78]

Lower or Prevent Insulin Resistance

Hormones play a major part in our health. Excess fat accumulation is often a result of an insulin spike which must be controlled through our eating habits and food choices. Insulin is a fat storage hormone. When we eat, insulin increases, signaling our body to store fat to use as fuel later. It's perfectly natural however persistently high levels of insulin leads to excess fat storage and

---

[7]https://www.ncbi.nlm.nih.gov/pmc/articles/PMC2562606/
[8]https://www.ncbi.nlm.nih.gov/pmc/articles/PMC3883043/

obesity, diabetes and many other issues. This is the main reason why people become overweight as opposed to the number or type of calories they consume.

Insulin is produced by the pancreas to allow our cells to absorb glucose to be used as a fuel source for energy. But certain cells become resistant to insulin, making them unable to absorb glucose effectively. This leads to a buildup of glucose within the bloodstream, and eventually pre-diabetes and diabetes.

Thankfully, you don't have to accept that insulin resistance and diabetes will be inevitable. Studies have found that with intermittent fasting you can greatly lower your blood sugar levels. Another study found that the practice of fasting is just as effective in treating insulin resistance as caloric restriction. Finally, not only can intermittent fasting prevent diabetes, but it can also treat diabetes when paired with the medical advice of a doctor, prevent blood sugar spikes and crashes, and increase the use and absorption of glucose.[9]

Lower Chronic Inflammation

Inflammation is a daily part of life and aids in keeping our body healthy. The immune system uses inflammation in order to treat injuries and prevent infections. Yet, some people develop high levels of inflammation which may become chronic. These cases of chronic inflammation are becoming more widespread with the modern diet, lack of sleep, too much work, and the stress of modern living. While inflammation may be a beneficial and

---

[9]https://www.sciencedirect.com/science/article/pii/S095528630400261 X

necessary component of our immune system when used in moderation, when it is increased in this way it becomes dangerous. Not only does increased levels of inflammation increase sleeping difficulties, pain, and many other symptoms, it can also increase the risk of disease. Studies have found chronic inflammation levels can lead to cancer, rheumatoid arthritis, heart disease, and more.

Thankfully, intermittent fasting has been shown to help resolve these problems. By following a fasting schedule for one month, participants within a study were able to lower their inflammation levels greatly. Another study found the same results when people practice daily twelve-hour fast for a month.[1011]

Increase your Brain Cells

Obviously, our brain cells are incredibly important. As we all know, we are unable to survive without our brain. Neurodegenerative diseases such as Alzheimer's and Parkinson's have increased in recent years. It has been found that our brain cells can often become damaged and stunted over time. Yet, studies have found that we can increase the growth of healthy brain cells and nerve tissue with the process of intermittent fasting. This, therefore, decreases the risk of neurodegenerative diseases developing later in life, may help treat any neurological diseases we have already developed, stabilizes mood, increases brain performance, and boosts both our focus and memory.

---

[10]https://www.sciencedirect.com/science/article/pii/S0271531712001820

[11]http://www.nrcresearchpress.com/doi/abs/10.1139/h09-014#.XEJguH2YWUk

Intermittent fasting has specifically been shown to increase cell growth within the hippocampus, basal forebrain, cortex, and nervous system due to triggering the brain-derived neurotrophic factor.[121314]

Repair Your Cells

Intermittent fasting has been shown to increase autophagy. This is a critical role within our bodies which help replace our old and decaying cells with younger and healthy cells. The point of this is to keep our bodies functioning in a homeostatic state. If autophagy isn't active enough, then we can develop diseases. The process is so powerful that researchers are searching for a way to increase autophagy with drugs, to help treat people with chronic and terminal diseases. By intermittent fasting you can increase this vital process naturally, helping to increase your lifespan and lower your risk of developing diseases. Studies have even found that it can help your stem cells activate into a state of self-regeneration.[1516]

Reduces Damaging Oxidative Stress

We commonly develop oxidative stress through our environment, food, lack of sleep, and even though the process of transmuting food into fuel and energy. When we develop oxidative stress and

[12]https://www.sciencedirect.com/science/article/pii/S156816370600052 3
[13]https://jneuroinflammation.biomedcentral.com/articles/10.1186/1742-2094-11-85
[14]https://onlinelibrary.wiley.com/doi/full/10.1046/j.1471-4159.2002.01085.x
[15]https://www.tandfonline.com/doi/abs/10.1080/15548627.2015.10637 68
[16]https://www.tandfonline.com/doi/abs/10.4161/auto.6.6.12376

free radicals it travels throughout our bodies and damages healthy cells. This in turns leads to disease and an increased rate of aging. However, we can combat the process. Studies have found that by practicing intermittent fasting, we are able to reduce oxidative stress and increase the antioxidants that fight against it. [17][18]

As you can see, there are many reasons to take up intermittent fasting. It may be scary to try something new, but study after study has proven not only its safety but its effectiveness as well. Fasting has historically been used for thousands of years to increase our health, and we now have science to back up all of its claims. Why hold back from something that could have such a powerful positive effect on your well-being?

Chapter 2:

Common Myths About Fasting

---

[17]https://www.sciencedirect.com/science/article/pii/S1568163706000523

[18]https://www.sciencedirect.com/science/article/pii/S0271531712001820

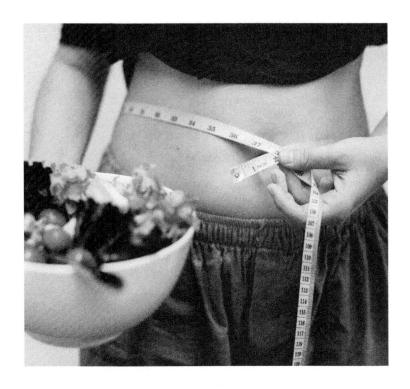

No matter what type of eating plan you start, there will always be criticizers who call it too tough or harmful. That's why it's important to have all the information before you begin and to debunk many common myths. We're taking some of the common myths about intermittent fasting and debunking them below

You're Starving Yourself

You are going to feel hungry at first as your body adjusts to a longer period without food – that's only natural. But, having your body adapt to change in diet is what causes physical changes like weight loss and health benefits. There is a stark difference in going without needed nutrition and choosing not to eat during a specific time period while still eating when needed. When you're deciding to fast, you're voluntarily restricting your calories, and you have the reassurance that at the end of your fasting window you will be able to eat. Intermittent fasting is all about timing. By extending the amount of time you are going without food, your body's hormones and metabolism begin to change in order to encourage weight loss.

You Need to Eat Small Meals

Actually, you don't. Intermittent fasting is about the quality of calories you're taking in when you are eating so that you can make it through the fasting window. When you are eating a diet with enough calories, you then have the energy to last through the fasting period and will not need to have a snack or a meal. Eating some small meals might help you feel better in the short term, as they soothe your growling stomach, but it won't help you gain the health benefits of fasting or spur on weight loss. It could do the opposite and increase your caloric intake and have your weight loss stop. That only helps when you extend your window of time without food and allow your body to burn fat it has stored away.

The Human Body Can't Survive Without Water

This is true, and that's why when you are fasting, you are encouraged to up your water intake, so you don't become dehydrated. If you want to fast for a long period of time, having enough water will help you do that, and other beverages like coffee or tea will give you a more filling effect. If plain water isn't enough for you, try infusing your ice cubes with some low-calorie fruit or mint in order to give your water more flavor. Remember, you can also have beverages so long as you are not taking them with cream or artificial sweeteners. Those "empty calories" might seem like nothing, but believe me they can add up

Your Brain Won't Get Enough Glucose

Many people are misguided in the belief that your brain will be deprived of glucose when you fast, but once again, that just isn't true. Your brain does need glucose, but a window of time without food doesn't mean your brain will be deprived of energy. When you skip a meal and are not having an intake of carbohydrates, your brain will get energy from ketones of fat molecules instead of glucose from carbohydrates. They are a great energy-rich fuel, and studies show that they actually improve cognitive functioning.

If I Don't Eat, I'll Lose Lean Muscle

I was concerned about this but there is no need to be. This is another myth where people think that participating in intermittent fasting will suddenly cause your muscles to shrink and disappear. That's just not true. After you eat a meal, your body is working hard to break down that food into molecules it uses for energy. It processes proteins, fats, and carbohydrates to store away. After it's used the meal for fuel, what will it do for more energy if you've decided to skip your next meal? We can assure you it doesn't turn on your muscles. It will instead turn to fat reserves it has stored away as energy and uses those to power you through the day.

A fasting window of anywhere from 12 to 20 hours is not enough time for an athlete to lose their muscles. The general rule of thumb is that fasting for a period of 48 hours or longer can be harmful. But, a short span of missing a meal or two does not have detrimental effects on the body's muscle mass.

Another truth that discounts this myth is that it takes a long time for the protein to be fully digested and absorbed by the body. It takes your body approximately six hours to burn off the protein of three eggs at the rate of 2.9 grams of protein an hour. If you drink a protein shake with twenty-six grams of soy protein powder, then it will take you approximately seven hours to absorb the protein at a rate of 3.9 an hour. Different protein sources are absorbed at different rates, between 1 and 10 grams of protein an hour depending on the source. As you can see, if you eat a large amount of protein before your fast, it can fuel you through either all or more of your entire fast!

Ah! But aren't Small Meals Supposed to Increase Metabolism?

This is a common myth, that is again, not true. People believe that the more you eat during the day, your metabolism will increase with each small meal. Yes, your body has to expend more energy to digest every small meal that you're eating, but that energy depends on the total calories you eat, not how many times a day you eat. So, eating 4 different three-hundred calorie meals will expend the same energy as eating two six-hundred calorie meals. The frequency of your meals will not impact how many calories you burn. The only way you will be calorie deficient enough to actually lose weight is by taking in fewer calories than you are expanding. By eating less and including exercise in your diet, your body will need to burn fat for energy to keep up with you. That's when real weight loss occurs. If you're stuffing yourself with empty calories throughout the day, your blood sugar will rise each time, and that can lead to more health conditions.

You'll Binge Eat After Fasting and Gain Weight

If you do intermittent fasting properly, you won't gain weight. This is only true if you overeat when you aren't fasting. It all depends on your individual behavior. You just need to get used to the fasting routine, and your appetite may even diminish as you continue with it.

To help yourself not binge eat after you finish fasting, you can practice by starting your fast gradually. Don't immediately jump into a sixteen-hour fast. Instead, try skipping a meal when you are naturally not hungry or doing an overnight twelve-hour fast between dinner and breakfast.

Non-fasting calories just need to stay below the calories missed while fasting for you to lose weight. The key is to eat healthy filling meals when you aren't fasting, not ones that are loaded with unhealthy ingredients and excessive calories. Sure, you might end up eating a few hundred calories more to compensate for the "lost" calories during your fasting window, but that overeating amount is still less than what you would have eaten for a full day without fasting.

Protein is Needed in Small Doses Throughout the Day for Muscle Growth

This is another common myth that science has debunked. It used to be that athletes believed they had to constantly supply their body with protein throughout the day for their muscles to continue to grow after a workout. New, research has shown that muscle growth actually occurs in the hours after you work out. Eating protein throughout the day won't increase your muscle growth. You simply need to eat your recommended amount of protein during the hours you are not fasting. This could even be all in one meal, but it is usually easier to stagger your protein intake over a time frame. It's a bit easier on your stomach too.

Twelve Hours without Food is a Long Time; it's Half of the Day

When you see the number as individual hours, it can seem like a very long time and very hard to do. But the truth is, you might be fasting for twelve hours without even realizing it. Let's say you have dinner at seven in the evening and are strict with yourself about no snacking before bed. Then the next morning, you're busy with getting ready and getting the kids to school that you have a cup of coffee but don't have breakfast until almost seven. That means you've fasted twelve hours without even realizing it It's all about structuring your day around your individual schedule. For sixteen hours, you would bump up your breakfast time to more of a brunch time. Treat yourself to enough coffee and water or tea to keep yourself going, and then have your first meal around eleven in the morning. That's a sixteen hour fast. This a great method to get you started.

I'm Worried that Fasting will Affect my Athletic Performance!

Another common myth is that fasting will hurt athletes in their performance on the field or in their workouts. Yet, research shows that this is not true. Intermittent fasting does not interfere with your body's performance when done correctly. Sure, when you start your fasting period, you might feel weak or slow, but that's because your body is simply adjusting to the change. It would be the same way if you started a new diet plan or cut caffeine or sugar from your diet. Once your body realizes you're not eating a meal for energy, it begins to burn the fat molecules it has stored away for energy. With that burst of energy, you can exercise, train, and play just like you normally would. Keep in mind, intermittent fasting recommends a higher intake of water as well, so that there is no risk of dehydration.

Fasting May Damage my Overall Health

There's no way on Earth that I would do that to my body. We understand that the first conclusion people will assume about not eating is that your body is in trouble. Although, the science proves otherwise. Research and studies show that intermittent fasting has a variety of health benefits as were as discussing. Weight loss is an obvious physical result, but it can also control your blood sugar, lower your cholesterol, and give you higher mental functioning and clarity. As with any change in your diet, it's important you speak to your doctor first to make sure you're a healthy candidate to follow an intermittent fasting model and that you would not be harming your health.

We've provided you the truth when it comes to these common myths about intermittent fasting so you are informed about how fasting will affect you.

Chapter 3:

The Pros and Cons of Intermittent Fasting

Does Intermittent Fasting Suit YOU?

You're in good health	You have had eating issues in the past
You can manage stress	You are experiencing a stressful time in your life or you are hormonal
You have a healthy relationship wth food	
You can control your eating especially when you break the fast	You are preoccupied with food during the fast
You feel better during the fast!	You overeat once you break the fast

It is tough giving up food for a set amount of time and avoiding the temptation of the delicious foods around you. You might feel hungry in the beginning, and cranky as you wish you'd eaten more, or you have a busy day ahead of you and you wish you could grab a snack. But the reason why so many people have made intermittent fasting a part of their lifestyle is due to the health benefits they will gain. It's a temporary hardship today to gain the benefits of better health in the future. And the scientific research proves it. Delaying instant gratification will benefit you in many ways, not just when it comes to food.

Here's some information regarding the health benefits and the potential cons of intermittent fasting.

The Positives of Intermittent Fasting:

You Can Lose Weight More Quickly

This is the obvious health benefit of intermittent fasting, but it's important to point out first. If you aren't finding much success in other diets or you feel like you're at a weight loss plateau and you're not able to get rid of some stubborn weight, intermittent fasting could be just what you need to speed up your weight loss. By telling your body there are certain windows of time you can eat, and windows of time when you cannot eat, you are lowering your caloric input. Being calorie deficient is what engages the body to start burning fat and losing weight. And because you don't have to count calories or macronutrients or divide up your diet into separate categories, a lot of people find fasting easier than alternative diets.

Studies have found that intermittent fasting is more effective than many other diet plans because it reduces the number of calories the body is intaking, and also increases the body's metabolic rate. As long as you aren't substituting the skipped meals with unhealthy meals or gorging on junk food, you should be on your way to losing unhealthy body fat. [19][20][21]

Intermittent Fasting Decreases Stress Hormones, and Increases Sleep Hormones at Bed Time

Melatonin is what the body naturally produces to help you fall asleep and stay asleep in order to get a good night's rest. Many people in today's society are sleep deprived, which affects not only their mood and wakefulness but also their weight loss. Intermittent fasting actually helps to release more melatonin at the correct time of night, so that your body can improve its sleep quality.

Cortisol is the stress hormone which can lead to symptoms such as weight gain, anxiety, fatigue, and insomnia when levels are too high in the body. Intermittent fasting works to reduce the level of cortisol in the bloodstream because your blood sugar is more regulated. If you have a sugary snack or eat a meal loaded with carbohydrates, your body's blood sugar rises, and cortisol is released into the bloodstream as the body panics at the sugar

[19] https://nutritionj.biomedcentral.com/articles/10.1186/1475-2891-11-98

[20] https://onlinelibrary.wiley.com/doi/full/10.1111/j.1467-789X.2011.00873.x

[21] https://www.sciencedirect.com/science/article/pii/S193152441400200X

hike. When you are fasting, there are less blood sugar spikes in the body which means less cortisol is being released. [222324]

Increase Heart Health and Lower Bad Cholesterol

Cholesterol is composed of multiple components. The main aspects of cholesterol are LDL (Low-Density Lipoprotein), also known as the "bad" cholesterol, and HDL (High-Density Lipoprotein), which is the "good" cholesterol.

Too high of an LDL level can be a factor of heart disease and potentially lead to a heart attack or stroke. Studies on obese individuals have shown that intermittent fasting can reduce cholesterol, LDL "bad" cholesterol, and the number of triglycerides in the cholesterol1. Triglycerides are fatty acids that cholesterol is composed of. This means that by decreasing the triglycerides, the cholesterol can become less harmful.

Intermittent fasting can also decrease blood pressure. This is because as the body burns fat molecules called ketones produced by the liver for energy when you're fasting, the liver has no time to secrete LDL too. It's providing you energy instead of producing a harmful substance.[2526]

[22]https://www.nature.com/articles/ejcn201332
[23]https://www.ncbi.nlm.nih.gov/pmc/articles/PMC5483233/
[24]http://jcsm.aasm.org/viewabstract.aspx?pid=28375
[25]https://www.karger.com/Article/Abstract/100954
[26]https://www.sciencedirect.com/science/article/pii/S0955286304002601X

Potentially Lowers the Risk of Developing Cancer

Although more studies need to be conducted on humans, many research studies on animals have shown that intermittent fasting could potentially prevent cancer. A study on rats showed that rats with tumors who were placed on dietary restrictions survived for longer than their counterparts who did not have any restrictions of food. This, among many other studies, suggests that intermittent fasting could inhibit cancer growth and increase the chances of survival. A study on human test subjects with cancer found that fasting reduced the side effects they felt from chemotherapy such as fatigue, weakness, and nausea. [27][28]

Fasting Increases Mental Alertness and Efficiency

Intermittent fasting raises the body's alertness by secreting a chemical called norepinephrine, or adrenaline. This is a neurotransmitter that gives the body focus and energy and is known to increase mental alertness. In rats, it was found that intermittent fasting creates new neural cells and connections between cells in the brain. That means neural signals can communicate and be processed faster to increase mental activity. Fasting has also been found to increase the presence of a brain hormone called brain-derived neurotrophic factor (BDNF). Lower levels of this hormone have been linked to mental illnesses such as depression and anxiety. It might seem counterintuitive that abstaining from food will actually increase mental alertness but

[27]https://www.nature.com/articles/pcan201024
[28]https://www.ncbi.nlm.nih.gov/pmc/articles/PMC2815756/

think about how eating a big meal makes you feel lethargic and lazy. When you are fasting and going without food, you will feel the opposite effects and feel more alert. Numerous studies have found that intermittent fasting does not decrease sleep, physical activity, or cognitive performance. [29][30]

It May Lengthen Your Lifespan

Though it's hard to tell without sufficient research on human test subjects, experiments on rats have found that intermittent fasting extended the lifespan of test groups that reduced their calories as opposed to the test group that did not change their diet plan. Even with having a heavier body weight, the fasting rodents actually lived longer than the control group. It could be because fasting improves the health of your immune system which could allow you to live longer. Many people use this as motivation for fasting. They can give up the comfort of food today in order to have a richer and longer life and spend that time with their family and friends. A temporary sacrifice now means a more important gain in the future.

Fasting Makes Life Easier and Simple

We're all busy people, and sometimes dealing with the hassle of getting breakfast or lunch in your busy day can seem like a hassle. This is especially true when you are on a diet. You might end up skipping meals because of how busy you are, and you just don't have the time to prepare a meal or get something to eat. Or if you

---

[29]https://www.sciencedirect.com/science/article/pii/S016517811200815 3
[30]https://www.sciencedirect.com/science/article/pii/S03069877070046 28

are too busy, you end up getting fast food or binge eating on unhealthy junk food instead.

When you make the decision to fast, you don't have to worry about meal prep or where to go for a last-minute quick meal. Instead, you can naturally feel satisfied until your normal eating window, as fasting becomes a habit and your body adjusts.
By powering through that time and keeping yourself busy, you'll have increased your fasting window. It's much easier than following a complicated diet plan where you might have to count calories, prepare pre-packaged meals, or buy protein shakes. Instead, there's no headache about what to cook and how you're skipping a meal because that's the entire point That's one less meal you have to shop for, cook and prepare, and clean up after Instead, by sticking to your fasting model, you can fit it into your schedule, so you are fasting when you are busy and then creating healthy meals when you have time.

The Negatives of Intermittent Fasting:

It May Be Difficult to Begin

A negative regarding intermittent fasting is that it tends to have a very high dropout rate. That's because it can be a very tough approach to adapt if you don't have the willpower to follow through or the knowledge to know how to begin. We are used to getting rewards or "cheat days" on our diets and feeling proud after we've done some hard work. But, depriving ourselves of food and drink makes those things even harder to achieve. Not to mention that your hormones and hunger pangs are in full effect when you're first depriving yourself of food. This is especially difficult when a person doesn't fully understand how to begin intermittent fasting. They may jump into a sixteen hour fast without ever previously fasting. The stark change is difficult to adjust to, leading them to feel like it's too hard or that they're a failure. If you begin slowly and use the tools you learn within this book you absolutely will succeed.

It Could Lead to Overeating

This is a common negative effect of intermittent fasting because people tend to overeat to make up for the "lost" calories on their fasting days or fasting window. Even if a person is physically full after a meal, mentally they might feel like they need to eat more because they were "starving" all day yesterday. When in fact, they were fasting. This destroys the purpose of intermittent fasting and may cause you to not lose the weight you wanted to.

This largely happens because the body is used to a certain number of calories, even if it's too much for your body type. Your body has learned to think that it requires a high caloric intake. But, if you control your urges to overeat, you can retrain your body into learning how much is an appropriate food intake.

Increased Hunger May Lead to a Hormone Imbalance

Leptin is the hormone that makes you feel full after you have eaten a meal. When you are undergoing intermittent fasting, your body's level of this hormone becomes imbalanced because you are hungry. This causes a hormone imbalance of leptin. Studies show that a severe imbalance in hormone levels could cause health problems in the future.

However, this hormone imbalance is usually rather mild, and it doesn't take long to recover from. Before long, your leptin levels should go back to normal.

You Might Become Dehydrated

This is critical, especially for people who already don't drink enough water but are tempted to fast to get quick weight loss results. When you are fasting, your cells are undergoing a metabolic process in a very quick amount of time. They need water to fuel these processes and give the cells strength. If you're not drinking enough water on top of fasting, then you could become severely dehydrated.

Not only that, but you tend to lose water weight when you are fasting. This means that your body is dumping much of its hydration. It's vital to replenish this hydration with more water. But of course you can drink coffee, tea, and calorie-free flavored water, as well.

Intermittent Fasting is not for Everyone

As we mentioned above, health issues could stop someone from fasting even if they really wish to attempt it. People with metabolic issues, severe diabetes, or those who are pregnant and lactating should also not try this method of weight loss because it could worsen their health. Some women also tend to have a very sensitive hormone balance, and this could cause damage to those levels. Intermittent fasting is also not recommended for teenagers who are still undergoing puberty and hormonal changes.

If you are considering fasting talk it over with your doctor and begin slowly with short fasts.

Chapter 4:

Intermittent Fasting for Treating Illness and Better Health

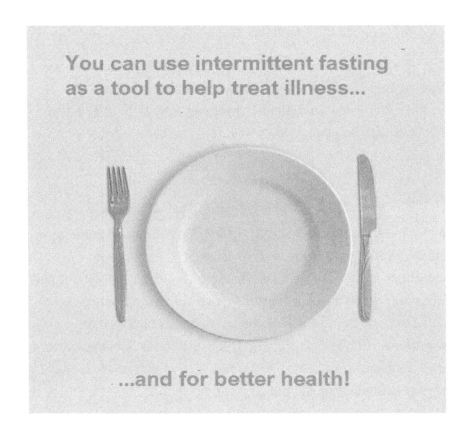

You can use intermittent fasting as a tool to help treat illness...

...and for better health!

Blood
Elevated keytone levels
Reduced glucose,, leptin
and insulin levels
Elevated idiponectin levels
Reduced inflammatory
keytones
Reduced markers of
oxiditive stress

Liver
Glycogen depletion
Keytone production
Increased insulin sensitivity
Reduced lipid
accumulation

Decreases
 Free radical damage
Weight gain and metabolic
desease risk
Triglyceride levels
decreasing risk of heart
desease

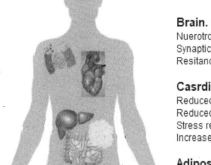

Brain. Improved Cognition
Nuerotrophic factor production
Synaptic plasticity
Resitance to injury and desease

Casrdiovascular system
Reduced blood pressure
Reduced resting heart rate
Stress resistance
Increased parasympathetic tone

Adipose tissue
Lipolysis
Reduced leptin production
Reduced inflammation

Muscle
Increased insulin sensivity
Enhanced endurance
Reduced inflammation

Intestines
Reduced inflammation
Enhanced mobility

Not only can intermittent fasting be used for weight loss, decreased insulin resistance, and a potentially increased lifespan, but it can also be used in order to treat disease. I must stress again that It's important always to discuss your dietary lifestyle with your doctor. This is especially true when you have a disease and are chronically ill. If you are hoping to use intermittent fasting in order to treat your symptoms and illness, then please discuss the details with your doctor beforehand. Within this chapter, we will go over some of the illnesses that intermittent has been shown to treat and manage.

Epilepsy

Before we had anticonvulsant drugs on the market and even before the century-long ketogenic diet was used to treat epilepsy, there was fasting. Ever since intermittent fasting was introduced for the treatment of epilepsy, it has been a viable option, especially when paired with the ketogenic diet. Both of these processes increase ketones and the mitochondrial cells, in the process protecting the brain from damage and decreasing the rate and intensity of seizures.

The ketogenic diet is widely known to help in the treatment of seizures. The ketogenic diet wasn't officially created until the early 1920s. Before then the dietary option for epilepsy treatment was regular fasting. This is because both of these approaches have a similar effect on brain chemistry, health, and our cells.

The benefits of fasting on epilepsy are first documented in studies in America and France in 1911. The study conducted in France placed twenty epileptic patients of different ages on a vegetarian low-carb diet paired with intermittent fasting. Some of the patients struggled with adjusting to the diet at first, but those who carried through with it experienced enormous benefits. They were able to not only decrease the number of seizures they were experiencing, but there were also able to increase their overall mental function. This was appreciated, as the medicines they were on at the time were known to dull mental functioning. Simultaneously, fasting was becoming well known within America for its treatment of epilepsy. Two of the main proponents of fasting were Bernnar McFadden and Hugh Conklin. Bernnar McFadden worked in the area if physical culture, a method that teaches combining strength training and diet for better health. He had found that fasting could control seizures and began popularizing the idea with researchers and doctors who decided to test the theory. Of these doctors was Hugh Conklin, a specialist in osteopathic medicine and a supporter of McFadden's.

Dr. Conklin treated hundreds of patients with uncontrolled epilepsy with the process of intermittent fasting. He would have them practice intermittent fasting for three to four weeks at a time. During this time his adult patients experienced a fifty percent rate of success and his adolescent patients a ninety percent rate of success. Combining all of his patients, fifty-percent were able to experience improvement and twenty-percent were able to become seizure free completely.

Not long later, Dr. H. Rawle Geyelin, a prominent endocrinologist from the New York Presbyterian Hospital, decided to recreate Dr. Conklin's work. During this process, he placed thirty-six patients on an intermittent fasting schedule, where he also experienced great results. These results were soon reported to the American Medical Association, which lead to a wider understanding of the benefits of fasting in the treatment of epilepsy. Another effective treatment for Epilepsy is CBD Hemp Oil which also has many other health benefits. I've used CBD Oil extensively and I'll share my experiences with this miraculous natural compound later in this book.[31][32]

---

[31]https://www.sciencedirect.com/science/article/pii/S0920121112003221
[32]https://onlinelibrary.wiley.com/doi/full/10.1046/j.1528-1157.2001.17601.x

Alzheimer's Disease

Alzheimer's disease is an incredibly prevalent and disruptive disease. This disease leads people to forget all about themselves and their loved ones. It's incredibly painful for both those living with it and their loved ones. Yet, this heart-wrenching disease is on the rise. Not only is Alzheimer's disease the sixth leading cause of death within the United States, but it's also increased by one-hundred and twenty-three percent between the years of 2000 and 2015. This is even more startling when you realize that scientists still do not understand the causes of Alzheimer's disease and why it's on the rise.

Thankfully, scientists have discovered some of the contributing factors of the disease. By focusing on these factors, we may be able to lessen the severity and commonality of the disease. One of the many factors in Alzheimer's disease is mitochondrial dysfunction, as well as a variation in a protein gene, immune system dysfunction, brain cell dysfunction, and more. Before long, these factors cause an increase in plaque and tangles of neurofibrillary within the brain. This process leads to oxidative stress, chronic inflammation, and further mitochondrial dysfunction. As you can see, this creates a vicious cycle where each process causes the next until it circles back on itself all over again.

Alzheimer's disease and its many components are known to lead to the neurons within the brain becoming resistant to insulin. As they become more resistant, they are unable to absorb the glucose they need to survive, ending in the brain cells dying. Thankfully, intermittent fasting has been shown to not only treat mitochondrial cell dysfunction but insulin resistance as well. This means that by incorporating intermittent fasting, you can reduce your risk of developing the disease and potentially even lessen the symptoms for people already living with it. [3334]

Parkinson's Disease

Parkinson's disease is one of the many neurodegenerative diseases that greatly affects a person's life. It can lead to cognitive impairment, difficulty moving, tremors, rigidity, chronic pain, slurred speech, fatigue, and depression. While the cause of this debilitating chronic disease is unknown, it has been found that a dysfunction of the mitochondrial cells is present and affects the condition. This dysfunction results in a large amount of oxidative stress and free radicals, which results in the symptoms commonly experienced. The damage is known to especially affect our brain cells that produce dopamine, not only causing depression but a wide range of issues. If this weren't bad enough for the sufferers of the disease, the common drugs used in treatment often becoming increasingly less effective while the negative side effects only increase.

Thankfully, intermittent fasting has been shown to decrease oxidative stress and heal the mitochondrial cells, directly combating the known issues surrounding Parkinson's disease. With intermittent fasting, a person may help ease their symptoms and slow the progression of their disease. [34]

Diabetes

---

[33]https://www.sciencedirect.com/science/article/pii/S0969996106003251
[34]https://www.pnas.org/content/97/10/5440.short

When you have extreme diabetes, you may not be able to practice intermittent fasting; this is because your condition may already be too severe to jump into this method of treatment. However, if you discuss your diabetes with your doctor, you can learn if it's a safe option to consider. Many people have found intermittent fasting to be a beneficial treatment option. This is largely due to the ability of intermittent fasting to treat insulin resistance and control weight.

A recent study published in 2018 found that intermittent fasting was highly effective for patients with type II diabetes who were insulin-dependent. Under their doctor's close eye these participants practiced twenty-four hour long fasts multiple times a week. With this treatment plan, there were able to reverse their insulin resistance, stop their medicine under their doctor's orders, and control their blood sugar levels. As if that weren't positive enough, the patients were also able to lower their body weight and stomach fat greatly.[35][36]

Cancer

A recent study on mice found that when they were on a diet that mimics fasting that chemotherapy was more effective in targeting skin cancer and breast cancer. Not only that, but the study found that while the immune system was able to better target the dangerous cancer cells, it was also able to better protect the healthy cells. This is incredible news, as chemotherapy is notorious for being an immunosuppressant. Researchers are

[35]https://www.sciencedirect.com/science/article/pii/S193152441400200 X
[36]https://febs.onlinelibrary.wiley.com/doi/full/10.1016/j.febslet.2007.02 .006

excited, because not only does this offer additional treatment for those who have cancer, but it's also inexpensive, feasible, and safe.

Another study tested intermittent fasting both prior to chemotherapy doses and afterward. The purpose of this study wasn't to assess its effectiveness, but rather its safety. Therefore, it was tested for a variety of lengths of time and on different types of cancers. A total of ten people participated, and fasting was found to be a safe treatment option in conjunction with chemotherapy.

But, how does this work? Studies have found that fasting can starve cancer cells and increase the effectiveness of chemotherapy. This is partially because cancer and tumor cells are only able to survive off of glucose for fuel. But this new study also found that its effects are because fasting increases important cells found within our bone marrow. The T and B cells are part of our immune system, and by increasing the number of these cells, they are able to directly target tumors and break them apart.[37][38]

Polycystic Ovary Syndrome (PCOS)

One of the most common endocrine disorders is polycystic ovary syndrome, often simply known as PCOS. This condition causes obesity, insulin resistance, fatigue, abnormal menstrual periods, infertility, increased growth of body hair, and more. Yet, this condition is one of many others where we do not yet know its

---

[37]https://news.usc.edu/103972/fasting-like-diet-turns-the-immune-system-against-cancer/
[38]https://www.ncbi.nlm.nih.gov/pmc/articles/PMC2815756/

cause. All the same, it is believed that excessive insulin, chronic inflammation, and genetics may impact this disease.

At this time there still needs to be more studies conducted on PCOS and inflammation. However, research suggests that when a person follows intermittent fasting regularly with a focus on healthy nutrition, they may experience beneficial results. They may especially notice an improvement in insulin resistance. While the research on intermittent fasting and PCOS is limited, there are more studies on the ketogenic diet and PCOS. This is relevant because the process of ketosis mimics fasting in many ways, especially with how the mitochondrial cells and insulin response. Therefore, positive results of the ketogenic diet lead to a valid hypothesis that intermittent fasting may be equally as effective in treatment.

In one study people with PCOS on the ketogenic diet were able to greatly improve their body weight, insulin resistance, and even infertility. A similar study in which the people were on a low-carbohydrate diet they experienced reduced insulin resistance, improved hormone balance, and increased fertility. Multiple studies have even found that people who had previously been infertile have been able to become pregnant once beginning a ketogenic diet.[39]

Multiple Sclerosis

Multiple sclerosis is a debilitating neurodegenerative disease which is known to cause an array of symptoms, including

[39]https://www.researchgate.net/publication/317858823_Fasting_as_po ssible_complementary_approach_for_polycystic_ovary_syndrome_Ho pe_or_hype

difficulties with movement, balance, memory, vision, and more. However, one study conducted by a team of the United States and Italian researchers found that intermittent fasting can reduce similar symptoms as well as enriched gut bacteria in mice. Due to the success, the researchers then moved on to testing intermittent fasting on sixteen people with relapsing multiple sclerosis. Not only did these participants experience the same benefits as the mice had, but they also developed a positive change of inflammation within their blood levels. This study is now being funded to go a step further, and forty people with multiple sclerosis are being tested on the effectiveness of intermittent fasting.

Another controlled and randomized study on forty-eight people with the disease studied the difference of the ketogenic diet and intermittent fasting. The participants experienced decreased inflammation, increased brain cell health, and improved memory. These benefits were seen equally both in the people on the ketogenic diet and those practicing intermittent fasting. This leads researchers to believe that when the two plans are combined together, they may be even more effective.[40]

Non-Alcoholic Fatty Liver Disease

Non-alcoholic fatty liver disease is a common condition in people who have an excessive amount of stomach fat. Some people may not even be overweight or have all that much stomach fat, but their body is predisposed to collecting fat within the liver. This is dangerous because if left untreated it may lead to liver failure and

[40]https://www.nationalmssociety.org/About-the-Society/News/Intermittent-Fasting-Changes-Gut-Bacteria-and-Redu

the need for a transplant. But, not only does intermittent fasting help increase weight loss and therefore fat within the liver, but it also directly targets the way the body stores fat. While a person with fatty liver disease is more likely to store fat within their liver than someone without it, scientists found that intermittent fasting can change this.

After targeting a specific protein gene, they were able to find that when this gene is higher within our bodies, our livers are less likely to hold onto excessive fat. The good news is that fasting naturally increases this protein gene, known as the 'growth arrest and DNA damage-inducible. This is extremely encouraging in the treatment of fatty liver disease, especially for those who are already at a healthy weight yet still their livers hold onto fat.[41]

Increased Mood

Mental disorders are much more common than people believe. Yet, over forty-million Americans (one in five) have a mental illness. One of the most common mental illnesses is depression, which is the leading cause of disability in young and middle-aged Americans. Sadly, two-thirds of the people with depression never seek treatment.

Thankfully, studies are showing that intermittent fasting can be powerful in managing depressive symptoms. Studies have found that within a week of beginning intermittent fasting people often experienced increased well-being, improved mood, increased alertness, tranquility, and even euphoria

[41]https://www.sciencedaily.com/releases/2016/05/160509085347.htm

Chapter 5:

Different Intermittent Fasting Methods

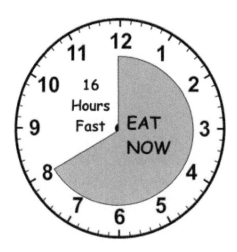

There are many different ways you can approach intermittent fasting as your daily or weekly routine. The flexibility these schedules provide is something that followers of fasting love because it's a simple formula that you can easily remember and adjust your day around. And you get to pick which method works best for you. It's entirely up to you what you can handle, what you can easily fit into your day, and what benefits you are seeing.

12/12 Method

This is a very simplistic method for beginners; you might even be doing twelve-hour fasts (or close to it) already without even realizing it. It's a great way to be aware of your eating habits and set your body to a rhythm of eating for only half the day. It's a good way to shorten your eating window in case you have an unhealthy habit of eating snacks after dinner. This method gives you twelve continuous hours of fasting, then an eating window of twelve continuous hours. It's a lot easier to do than you might think. Unless you are one of those midnight snacke-rs or you eat breakfast very early in the morning, a lot of people are fasting this amount of time or close to it.

(Example) Let's say you finish your dinner by 7:30 P.M. every night. You want to be sure that you had enough to eat and that you are firm with yourself that you will not eat anything afterward. Then the next day, even if you are an early riser, try to fill your time until 7:30 A.M. with coffee or water. Once 7:30 A.M. hits, you have completed your twelve-hour fast and can eat your breakfast. That means you've completed the 12/12 Method successfully.

16/8 Method

This is the most popular method for intermittent fasting, and it was made popular by fitness trainer Martin Berkhan who recommended this method. It is also referred to as the Leangains Method. This method follows a routine of 16 continuous fasting hours followed by an eight-hour eating window. This method can be tweaked for women. Men tend to have higher body mass index and can follow sixteen hours of fasting, while women should follow fourteen to fifteen hours. Then, their eating window can be from nine to ten hours. This method is very appealing to people who find it impossible to go a full day or more without food. Simply skipping one meal a day can do the trick for most people

You are probably sleeping for seven to eight hours anyway, and as we've said that time counts towards your fast.

This chart of the Leangains method is provided by James Clear: https://jamesclear.com/the-beginners-guide-to-intermittent-fasting

This method can be a little more difficult if you get hungry early in the morning, but you can always tweak the method and you're your dinner earlier so you can ensure a sixteen hour fast. Actually, most people who don't have breakfast are probably following this

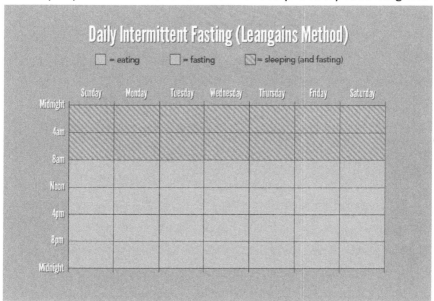

fasting method. It's really is quite easy to do. And don't forget, you can fill in that time before a meal with water or coffee to dull your growling stomach. When your eating window arrives, you want to be sure you fit in two healthy, filling meals or three smaller, healthy meals. If you end up gorging on junk food or unhealthy fats during your eating window, you just won't gain the health benefits. This method will push your body towards burning fat for energy.

A great way to follow this method is to skip breakfast and restrict your eating time so you can fit in a healthy lunch and dinner. If you finish eating dinner by seven, then you need to be sure you abstain from eating until around eleven. (or a little earlier if you're a woman and cutting your fast time by an hour or two). This would mean you have completed a sixteen-hour fasting window. Then from eleven to seven, you want to be sure you are planning to have two healthy, protein and energy-rich meals, along with a healthy snack or two. A lot of people find this kind of method convenient because they can fill their morning time with coffee or water until they hit their eating window. This allows people to enjoy eating meals with friends or family. Skipping breakfast is easy enough to do privately, but for lunch or an early dinner, you can still make plans to enjoy some company for the meal.

20/4 Method

If you've gotten comfortable with the 16/8 Method, this method turns things up a notch. This follows a method where you will fast twenty consecutive hours and allow for a four-hour eating window. You have to be sure to pace yourself with beverages during your fast window and fit in two healthy meals during the short eating window. You want to prepare meals with lots of proteins and carbs to ensure you have enough energy to get through that twenty-hour fasting window. Be sure you're drinking enough water and have a supply of caffeinated beverages to get you through any tough spots.

With only four hours to eat, you should fit that window during a time you can have two meals, like a late lunch and early dinner if your four-hour window is from three to seven. This means you can have a late lunch and plan to have a filling dinner to carry you until the next day. Be sure you eat your lunch right around three so you will be hungry by the time it's seven and time for dinner. You can even eat a healthy snack or two, like nuts, seeds, Greek yogurt, or an avocado. After dinner, you can have water or tea before bed and then be sure to keep yourself busy in the morning to make it to three. Caffeine should help you with this method.

5:2 Method

This method is also called the "Fast Diet." Michael Mosley, a British journalist, and doctor promoted this method of fasting as a way of living longer, losing weight, and looking younger. He even had a TV show on the BBC that made this method very popular to the general public. This method can be quite tough to undergo. It means a person will normally eat five days of the week and then restrict their calories to only five-hundred to six-hundred calories for two days of the week. Women are recommended to consume five-hundred calories on fast days, while men should have six-hundred calories since they tend to have a higher body mass index.

For this method, it's all about fasting on the days you find convenient. It might work better on a day when you know you will be very busy from morning to night, so you won't be noticing your hunger or tempted to unnecessarily snack. You might eat a normal diet every day except for Mondays and Saturdays where you are sure to limit your intake to five-hundred or six-hundred calories. That could mean two meals that are either two-hundred and fifty or three-hundred calories each depending on if you're male or female. Be sure that you have healthy food and protein sources stocked up and know exactly what you will eat that day, so you aren't wasting time or tempted to break your calorie restrictions. It's also important you count your calories, so you aren't going over your number in order for this method to be effective. The free online apps later in the book will help you track macro nutrients i.e. protein, carbs and fats as well as overall calories.

Eat Stop Eat Method

Fitness expert Brad Pilon made this method very popular in the year 2000. This method requires a full twenty-four hour fast once or twice a week. You can fill that twenty-four-hour time period with non-caloric drinks, coffee, and tea, but you should abstain from any solid food. You can try calorie-free gum too, which will fool your stomach for a little while that you're getting sustenance. But it does sound pretty daunting, right? It can require a lot of self-discipline, and you want to be sure you've "worked your way up" from the other methods we mentioned before, so your body is properly trained to undergo this challenge. It can be very difficult, and it's not for everyone, and there's no shame in admitting that

You could follow this method by fasting from after breakfast one day to breakfast time the next day. Or if you prefer having dinner, you could start your fast after dinner then skip your meals and have plenty of beverages to tide you over until dinner the next night. A good idea is to allow your fast days to fall when you know you will be very busy from morning to night. The busier you are in your day, the less focused you will be on your feelings of hunger.

Example: to follow this method, you could have dinner at eight on a Friday night then abstain from eating anything until eight on Saturday night. You want to be sure that you have enough beverages to "fill" you up, and that you have a busy schedule ahead of you on Saturday to keep you occupied. That will help make the time go by faster

Alternate Day Fasting Method

This method can also be quite tough to get into, so we recommend you work your way up to this level. This method means you are fasting every other day, though some methods do allow a minimum of around five-hundred or six-hundred calories depending on your gender (like we mentioned in the 5:2 Method). This method is usually undertaken by people who want to see serious weight loss results fast.

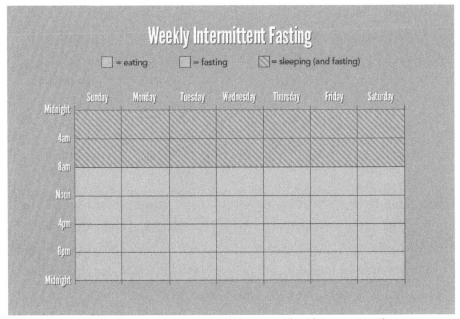

This chart of the Leangains method is provided by James Clear: https://jamesclear.com/the-beginners-guide-to-intermittent-fasting

This type of fasting with twenty-four hours with food then twenty-four hours without food can be quite tough to implement for a long period of time. It can actually be very hard to sustain. Studies on animals have shown that when they followed an alternate day fasting method, they would end up consuming twice the calories on the "on" days to make up for the fasting day. It can be quite extreme and unnecessary because following one of the other methods we've mentioned previously can still allow you to lose weight and improve your health.

This method is similar to the Eat Stop Eat method we mentioned previously, but you will have to be more rigid as you follow an alternate day pattern of fasting. You could have dinner on

Tuesday night, then fast until dinner on Wednesday night. After that, you will be sure to eat enough and increase your caloric output, and then start another twenty-four hours of continuous fasting after dinner on Thursday.

The Warrior Diet…. the what?

This diet became popular in 2001 when it was created by an ex-Israel Special Forces soldier named Ori Hofemkler. He transitioned his career to fitness and nutrition and coined the "Warrior Diet" based on patterns of eating that follow ancient warriors. It was created to improve how a person feels, eats, acts, and looks, and it follows the patterns of warriors of who ate very little during the day and feasted at night. It's similar to the 20/4 Method in the sense that you "fast" all day and then allow yourself to "feast" at night. Hofemkler and other followers of the diet claim that the Warrior Diet burns more fat gives an energy boost and improves mental clarity and concentration.

During the twenty-hour fasting window, you are encouraged to eat healthy fruits and vegetables, dairy products, nuts, and seeds, and be sure to have plenty of non-calorie fluids. Then when night falls, the "feast" period begins where you can eat foods of your choice. It's encouraged that you continue to eat healthy unprocessed foods to gain the most health benefits.

This diet also emphasizes a Paleo diet which consists of unprocessed, raw foods that mimic what they look like in their natural form. That means eating healthy, lots of raw fruits, vegetables, and nuts, and very little processed food.

To begin this diet, there is an initial three-week plan for beginners to get them comfortable with what they can and cannot eat.

(Hi again! What do you think of the book? Is it helping you? I would love if you could please take two minutes to leave me an honest review on this linkhttp://www.Amazon.com/gp/customer-reviews/write-a-review.html?asin=B07NQQY5TZ

Thank you! Robert.

Chapter 6:

Fasting and Working Out

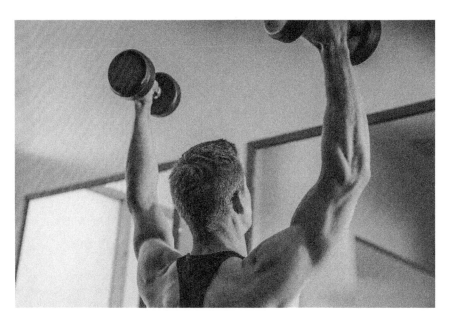

When we want to lose weight, we are often told to restrict our calories and greatly increase our exercise. This plan has its roots in reality, but it is often taken to an ineffective extreme that only further increases your struggles with weight loss.

Oftentimes, after feeling frustration at a lack of weight loss people will only further restrict their calories and increase their exercise, compounding upon the problem they don't even see that they have. Why? This is largely due to the hormones within our bodies. When we exercise and greatly restrict calories our leptin, cortisol, and ghrelin hormones signal to our brains that we must eat. This happens to such a degree that we can overeat without realizing it or without feeling that we can stop ourselves. The need to eat feels visceral, and due to that, we end up ruining our hard work. As if that weren't damaging enough, this process is known to raise levels of inflammation, speed up cell aging, and increase fatigue.

However, exercising doesn't have to be this way. When you exercise during a fasting period, you are able to gain all of the benefits of a tough workout but at a much more manageable intensity. You will find that you are losing more weight than you otherwise would, but without having to overdo it and push your bodies to extremes. This, in turn, will help your hormones stay balanced and prevent you from overeating later on.

While exercise can be greatly effective while in a fasted state, it's important that you listen to your body. If you are a high-intensity athlete, you may experience a slight decrease in your capabilities while fasted, but if you save your fasting for when you are not working out, then it shouldn't affect your performance or routine.

The reason for this is simple. Some types of exercise, those that make use of short bursts of high-intensity, require API energy, which requires glucose. This energy is stored within our muscles to help us when we suddenly become active. For instance, if you suddenly needed to run away from danger this glucose-derived API energy would help your muscles instantly adapt. But, if you haven't eaten carbohydrate, then you are unlikely to have the API energy you require to perform tasks such as bodybuilding or CrossFit at your previous intensity.

If you hope to perform high-intensity exercises while in a fasted state to increase your weight loss, then be sure to plan ahead and listen to your body. If you find yourself getting dizzy or light-headed, then you should slow things down and give your body a chance to recover. Remember, the longer the fast, the more likely you are to experience these symptoms. But, as long as you listen to your body and stay hydrated, you should be okay. It's also important to know that you are more likely to experience these side effects while you are still adjusting to fasting. Studies have shown that after people adapt to intermittent fasting, the entire process becomes easier, including exercising while you are fasted.

In order to plan ahead, you might want to eat an increased number of carbohydrates prior to your fast. The last meal before you begin your fast simply consume something such as whole-wheat pasta, sweet potatoes, beets, or other healthy options that can increase the amount of glucose-derived API energy within your muscles. This is often best to do the night before your workout so that you have enough energy to do high-intensity exercise but can still gain the weight loss benefit from exercising in the fasted state.

If you don't care for intense, all-out exercise, then the good news is that cardio is a wonderful ideal option while you are fasting. You are able to get the full benefits of exercising in a fasting state with cardio, but because it is not a high-intensity exercise it does not require API energy. Due to this, cardio can be especially helpful for people who are on a ketogenic diet while practicing intermittent fasting. These people won't need to be as careful about consuming enough carbohydrates in order to complete their workouts. Instead, they can maintain a low-carb lifestyle while being full of energy.

Cardio is especially powerful with intermittent fasting because you never want to practice it on a full stomach. If you try to do cardio immediately after eating, then the required blood flow for the muscles will interfere with the digestion process. This then prevents our bodies from being able to absorb all of the vital nutrients found within our meals. Therefore, be sure that you only practice your cardio after you have been fasting for a minimum of three to four hours.

Most people have been advised to fill up before a training session. Whether it's one of those pre-workout smoothies or eating a heavy protein-filled meal, this is advice that many people receive from their trainers. This is supposed to help you achieve the best work out you can. But new research has shown there are many health benefits to working out while fasting or without having eaten a large meal just before working out.

One major benefit is that your body becomes more sensitive to insulin. When you eat frequent meals throughout the day, the carbohydrates in your meal cause your blood sugar to spike. This means insulin has to work harder to carry those sugars around your body and stabilize your blood sugar again. The more frequently you have these spikes, the more resistant insulin becomes, and that can mean high blood sugar levels and a risk for Type II diabetes.

Martin Berkhan, who popularized the 16/8 fasting method (see Chapter 5) was able to promote his fasting plan on athletes and bodybuilders because of an experiment he did regarding fasting and working out. He did a study in 2010 where he had three groups:

- Group C: The group of male athletes in this group ate a carbohydrate-rich pre-workout meal before their training.
- Group F: This group practiced training while fasting. They received the same meal as Group C but ate it later in the day after working out.
- Control Group: The males in this group ate the same meal as the two previous groups but did not work out.

The study found that Group F that fasted while exercising and ate later in the day had better insulin sensitivity than Group C. They also had better glucose tolerance. This could be because they had less frequent meals throughout the day which allowed their body to have stable blood sugar throughout the day instead of constant spikes.

You secrete more growth hormone when you limit your meals. As we mentioned earlier, a longer fasting window means the body will secrete more human growth hormone or HGH. This hormone is responsible for maintaining bone density and muscle mass. Research has shown that frequent eating actually restricts the release of human growth hormone due to the glucose spikes in your system. A study in Science Daily found that fasting for twenty-four hours raised human growth production by almost two-thousand percent in men, and thirteen-hundred in women. Wow

Now, it's not necessary that you do a twenty-four hour fast, because that can be quite intense. But even delaying your first meal of the day after you work out can allow HGH to be secreted to help you get the most optimal workout and muscle growth.

Working out while fasting also increases testosterone production. Even women have small amounts of testosterone in their body as it pertains to issues like muscle mass and energy levels. Those are very important when it comes to giving you the energy you need when training

Many athletes say that they feel slower and lazier when they've just eaten a huge meal and then go straight to working out. They feel "sluggish" as if they are not able to perform to their best level because of their full stomach. By fasting, you're able to work out on an empty stomach and gain all the health benefits that come with a longer fasting window. That means your testosterone and HGH is secreting and working together to give you the best workout

Fasting before working out forces your body to shed fat. Fasting is a process that activates your sympathetic nervous system, along with exercise. This is the body's system that is responsible for

73

burning fat. This combination of fasting and exercising pushes the sympathetic nervous system to activate cellular catalysts and processes including the AMP Kinases and cyclic AMP, which break down stored fat reserves for energy. The body realizes it's not getting a "fresh" fuel source meal, so it uses what it has stored away.

One study found that eating before working out can decrease body weight but fasting can decrease both body weight and body fat. If you're more interested in getting rid of overall body fat and keeping that weight off, fasting would be the best method for you.

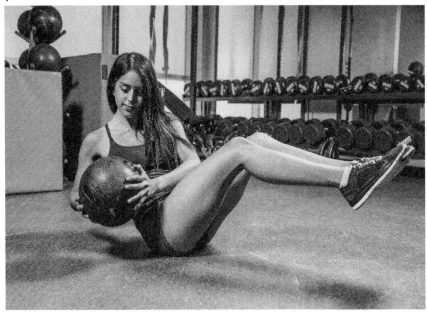

Exercising while fasting keeps your muscles and neurons biologically young. Together, fasting and exercises create a process of oxidative stress on the body, but this stressful process actually keeps your muscles young. It stimulates the cells to create antioxidants which allow for the cells to better resist fatigue and generate new energy. This counteracts signs of aging and gives new life to aging cells. This process occurs in muscle cells and neural cells.

So, what is the best way to gain the benefits of intermittent fasting and exercising combined? You have to adjust your fasting times to your workouts to ensure you're getting the optimal workout. Here are some options you can try

- Exercising first thing in the morning. If your target fast is anywhere from fourteen to sixteen hours (around fourteen for women, sixteen for men), that means only eating from about eleven in the morning to seven in the evening. Essentially, this means you can skip breakfast and make lunch your first meal of the day instead. By exercising when you are still fasting, you can get many of the health benefits we mentioned above. This will engage your sympathetic nervous system and ensure your body starts burning fats. You should feel rested after a good night's sleep and don't have to worry about a full stomach slowing you down, so you can get in a morning workout before your big brunch meal around eleven. Don't forget to stay well hydrated. That will ensure you have the energy you need.

- If your exercise consists of heavy weight lifting, it's important that you eat around thirty to sixty minutes after your work out so that your body can quickly accumulate protein. Unless of course you are simply not hungry after your workout albeit you probably will be. Always listen to your body. It's never wrong. Whey protein is a great option here and can also be a beneficial pre-workout meal if you're stuck for time. It's also important to get some easily-digested healthy carbohydrates, such as those from fruits or vegetables. You could make a whey protein shake and add in some frozen fruit or even a beet. Although, if you want you can always eat a sweet potato with some of your favorite healthy toppings that are rich in protein.

- Use your common sense. Many factors play a role into whether you can successfully exercise when fasting: your age, what your last meal was if you're taking medication, your level of fitness, the type of workout you're doing. A lot of things matter You are the best person who can determine how you are feeling when you are fasting and if you are able to exercise. If you feel weak and nauseous without food, then maybe you have to wait to exercise after your fasting window is finished. If you feel fine and feel like you have more energy on an empty stomach and don't feel as slow, then you can fit in an energetic workout and then look forward to breaking your fast with an energy-rich meal

There are many fantastic and free online tools which will absolutely benefit you. I find them invaluable and I use them daily to great effect. Measuring your progress is fun and will help you achieve your goals faster.

Here is a list of the best apps currently available. Have a look and see if there's anything you fancy. I would recommend starting with MyFitnessPal and go from there. Signing up is really simple and these apps are easy to use.

Fitness

1. Couch to 5K
(Free; iOS and Android)

2. Blogilates
(Free with optional in-app purchases; iOS and Android)

3. Sworkit
(Free with optional in-app purchases; iOS and Android)

4. Strava Running and Cycling
(Free with optional in-app purchases; iOS and Android)

5. Daily Yoga
(Free with optional in-app purchases; iOS and Android)

6. Nike+ Training Club
(Free; iOS and Android)

7. Endomondo

(Free with optional in-app purchases; iOS and Android)

8. MobilityWOD
(Free; iOS)

9. Aaptiv
(Free; iOS and Android)

10. SweatWorking
(Free; iOS)

11. Strong Workout Tracker Gym Log
(Free; iOS)

12. Sweat
(Free; iOS and Android)

13. Pear
(Free; iOS and Android).

Food and Nutrition

14. Foodility
(Free; iOS)

15. MyFitnessPal
(Free with optional in-app purchases; iOS and Android)

16. Lifesum
(Free with optional in-app purchases; iOS and Android)

17. Rise
(Free with optional in-app purchases; iOS)

18. Fooducate
(Free with optional in-app purchases; iOS and Android)

19. Nourishly
(Free; iOS and Android)

20. Oh She Glows
($1.99 with optional in-app purchases; iOS and Android)

21. Yummly Recipes + Shopping List
(Free; iOS and Android)

22. Waterlogged
(Free with optional in-app purchases; iOS and Android)

Mind and Brain

23. Meditation Studio
($2.99; iOS)

24. H*nest Meditation App
($1.99; iOS)

25. Talkspace
(Free with optional in-app purchases; iOS and Android)

26. Happify
(Free with optional in-app purchases; iOS and Android)

27. 7 Cups (Free; iOS and Android)

28. Wysa
(Free; IOS and Android)

29. Happy Not Perfect
(Free with optional in-app purchases; IOS and Android)

30. Grateful

(Free; IOS)

31. Pacifica
(Free with optional in-app purchases IOS and Android)

32. Awaken
(Free with optional in-app purchases; IOS)

33. Calm
(Free with optional in-app purchases; IOS and Android)

Overall Health

34. HealthTap
($99 per month), which allows you unlimited video and text chatting with doctors. (Free with in-app purchases; iOS and Android)

35. Sleep Cycle
(Free with in-app purchases on iOS, $0.99 on Android)

36. Power Nap App
(Free; iOS)

37. Leafly
(Free; iOS and Android)

38. Flo
(Free; IOS and Android)

39. SleepScore
(Free with optional in-app purchases; IOS and Android)

40. AmWell

The app is free, but the appointments start at $65 (or less, depending on insurance). (Free; IOS and Android)

41. Habitica
(Free; IOS and Android)

Chapter 7:

Eating Healthy, Energy-Rich Foods

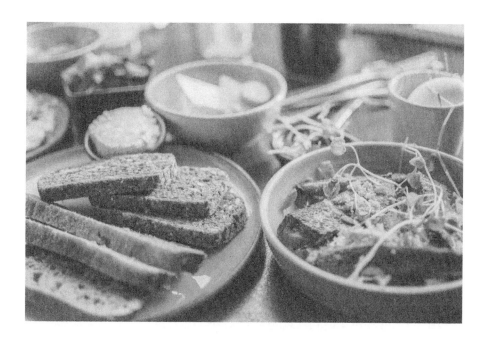

If you are going to be fasting for twelve to twenty-four hours of the day, you're probably wondering what you should eat to give you the energy needed to complete your fast. Eating a diet full of protein, fiber, and healthy fats, which are whole energy-rich sources of fuel is the only way to ensure you'll have success completing your fast. Ensuring you feel full throughout your fasting window will lower your hunger pangs and help you resist temptation.

Here are some great suggestions about what you should and shouldn't eat on an intermittent fasting schedule.

Fish

Fish is high in healthy fats, omega 3 fatty acids, and protein. It's considered "brain food" because omega 3 acids are considered vital in protecting the cell receptors of cell membranes. They help fight anxiety, depression, heart disease, inflammation, and more American Dietary Guidelines recommend at least eating 8 ounces of fish per week. Try including fish in your meals at least twice a week to ensure you get your protein along with the other important vitamins and minerals. However, there are many types of fish, and you may be wondering which are the best to choose from. In general, most fish are a good option. But there are some that are obviously better than others. We all know about the amazing properties of wild-caught salmon, which is one of the best fish options, so let's look at a couple of the other options.

While there are certainly people who are unable to get enough of sardines, the majority of people within the United States has rarely tried one and has no desire to do so. This is sad because sardines are one of the top fish options when it is packed in healthy options, such as olive oil. These fish are high in omega-3 fatty acids, calcium, selenium, vitamin D, and more. This helps them to support your overall health. The thing is, there is more to sardines than meets the eyes. Some fish can be high in heavy metal poisoning, and oftentimes the larger the fish, the higher level of mercury can be found within it. This is because larger fish eat smaller fish, and with each fish, they eat their level of mercury poisoning increases. When you eat the fish, you take on the level of mercury found within it. However, sardines are an incredibly small fish, and because of that, they are also really low in heavy metals.

Mackerel is a sustainable fishing option that is unlikely to cause any large degree of habitat destruction. Like sardines, this fish is also lower in heavy metal poisoning. A single three-ounce serving contains twenty grams of protein and is high in vitamin B12, selenium, magnesium, phosphorous, and potassium.

It is best to avoid bluefin tuna. Not only is this species incredibly overfished leading to putting it on the endangered species lists, but it is also high in heavy metal poisoning. Similarly, you should avoid imported mahi-mahi, Atlantic farm-raised salmon, and halibut wild-caught in the Atlantic.

Meat

If you're looking for a meal full of protein and fiber, red meat is the way to go. Beef, in particular, contains a lot of protein to ensure you feel energized throughout the upcoming fasting period and can complete all your workouts. Just one cut of steak contains approximately sixty-two grams of protein and can be filling enough to last you all day But, it's important that if you can afford to do so that you choose the highest sourced beef you can. While you may have to go with the cheap beef options, it is highly recommended to choose the antibiotic-free, organic, grass-fed options when you can afford it.

You most likely have heard "you are what you eat," and this phrase applies to what your food ate during its lifetime, as well. Because of this, the nutrition difference of grain-fed beef and grass-fed beef is significant.

Grass-fed beef is twice as high in the healthy conjugated linoleic acid. It's three times as high in the all-important omega-3 fats. And, it's also much higher in many other nutrients such as vitamins, minerals, and antioxidants.

Even more than sardines, organ meats are often overlooked in the Western developed world. While people often ate these meats out of necessity, with the rise of industrialized farming people began only buying select cuts of meats and therefore shunning those that were seen as something for the impoverished. But, not only is it economical to enjoy these cuts of meat, but it is also great for your health. The best example of organ meat is the liver, whether it comes from a cow, chicken, sheep, or another animal. This selection of meat is high in an incredible number of nutrients, including potassium, zinc, folate, thiamine, riboflavin, biotin, copper, phosphorous, iron, choline, and vitamins A, C, B12, D, and B6.

While most Americans rely on taking a multivitamin, these pills are not easily absorbed into the body. But, when you eat the nutrients in your food, such as in the liver, you are much more likely to reap the benefits.

Since organ meats have fallen out of favor, many people search for reasons to avoid it and lean further toward their standard choices. This has caused the spread of misinformation and myths on organ meats that are simply not true. For instance, people have come to believe that the liver holds onto all the harmful chemicals within the body and is therefore not safe to eat. They think that just like fish hold onto mercury that liver holds onto harmful compounds. But this is not true. The liver is not a sieve that catches the harmful compounds from the body and holds onto them. Instead, the liver removes and excretes these compounds, never holding onto them. The liver contains no more harmful compounds than any other piece of meat. Of course, if you want the best quality liver, you can choose organic, but if you are going to splurge on organic ingredients, it may be better to choose other cuts of meat or fruits and vegetables to spend that money on and instead just buy regular liver. Of course, if you can buy all of your food organic, then that is ideal. Also, using a slow cooker to make most meats will make it very soft, tender and tasty.

Eggs

I love eggs. I eat a lot of them! One large chicken egg alone can carry up to 6 grams of protein. They even cook in just a few minutes They may be small but are packed with protein which is important to keep you full while fasting and building muscle growth. Whether it's quick scrambled eggs or hard-boiled eggs, they cook quickly and are a great, filling meal or snack. Many studies show that people who tend to have eggs for breakfast stay feeling full until longer in the day.

But there are more eggs to choose from then just chicken eggs. While these are the standard, quail eggs are also incredibly healthy. These tiny eggs can be found at specialty health food grocery stores, farmers' markets, and Asian food markets. These eggs are a wonderful source of vitamins A, B1, B2, protein, and healthy cholesterol. Surprisingly, quail eggs contain fifteen times more B2 and six times more vitamin B1 than the larger chicken eggs. Quail eggs have also been shown to decrease allergies, increase metabolism, manage blood pressure, improve vision, boost energy, stimulate growth and cell repair, and even cleanse the body of harmful toxins. Even if you choose to mainly consume chicken eggs, you can greatly benefit by adding quail eggs to your diet a few times a week.

Legumes and Beans

Legumes and beans may be high in carbohydrates, but they are great protein sources that pack energy into your routine. This means that they will help you get through that fasting period. Plus, they are packed with fiber which allows you to feel full for longer and ensure you don't have any digestive issues. Beans such as chickpeas and black beans also tend to decrease body weight because they are a healthier protein source than red meat. If that weren't beneficial enough, they are known to lower total cholesterol levels, significantly reduce insulin, increase gut health, manage blood sugar, and more.

Some of the most nutrient-packed beans and legumes include chickpeas, lentils, kidney beans, peas, black beans, soybeans, pinto beans, navy beans, and peanuts. Yes, peanuts are a legume, not a nut.

Whole Grains

Whole grains are full of both fiber and protein, which again are two things which are very important in keeping you feeling full during your fasting window. Studies show that whole grains can even increase your metabolism which is great when you couple that with your intermittent fasting and exercise routines.

Sadly, many Americans have replaced whole grains with refined grains. While whole grains are a complete package of nutrition, refined grains have had this removed. This is because whole grains are made up of three components: bran, germ, and the endosperm. All three of these portions of the grain contain various nutrients such as fiber, vitamins, minerals, and phytonutrients.

You may have previously heard of fiber, vitamins, and minerals, but what are phytonutrients? Put simply these are natural and healthy chemicals found within all plants. While vitamins and minerals are incredibly important for our health, it now appears that many of the health-promoting benefits found within plants are a result of a rich assortment of phytonutrients.

These nutrients and their benefits are unable to be replicated within a pill. This means in order to attain the benefits of phytonutrients we must consume a large a varied diet full of a variety of plants.

Yet, when these grains are processed the incredibly healthy bran, and germ are removed, leaving only the quickly digested endosperm. This can cause blood sugar crashes and spikes because the fiber within the brain helps to stabilize blood sugar. The fiber is also important in lowering cholesterol, maintaining gut health, and preventing dangerous blood clots.

As you can see, removing the germ and bran which not only contain phytonutrients but also fiber is detrimental to your health. The germ is removed during the refining process because it contains healthy fats. But, while these fats are healthy, they shorten the shelf life of a product. Since manufacturers are mainly looking to make money, they want products that can sit on the shelves for ages without needing to be replaced with fresher products. But, the germ of the grain is one of the healthiest portions of the grain as it is high in phytonutrients, B vitamins, fiber, and vitamin E.

Studies have found that rather focusing on the number of grains you are eating; it's important to focus on the quality. This means that if you are only eating a few grains, but they are all refined you will not be gaining the same health as someone who focuses on eating whole grains such as whole wheat, brown rice, and millet.[42]

Vegetables

---

[42]https://www.hsph.harvard.edu/nutritionsource/what-should-you-eat/whole-grains/

Cruciferous vegetables such as cauliflower, broccoli, and brussels sprouts are full of fiber that will help your digestion stay regular and prevent constipation during your fasting period. As we stated above, the more fiber you eat, the fuller you will feel for longer which will motivate you during your 14 or 16-hour fasting window. This fiber will also better stabilize your blood sugar and lower your cholesterol.

These vegetables are also known to regularly contain vitamin K, C, and E, folate, a variety of minerals, carotenoids, and glucosinolates. While you may be unfamiliar with glucosinolates, this is an important phytonutrient that is responsible for the characteristic flavor and smell of cruciferous vegetables. This compound has been found to be incredibly important for the associated health benefits of cruciferous vegetables.

Along with cruciferous vegetables, you want to choose vegetables that are also high in fiber (we mention fiber a lot...we like fiber!) and nutrients to keep you full and energized. While lettuce may be a healthy option, a simple lettuce salad is not going to hold you over or offer a wide variety of nutrients your body requires.

Instead, if you are someone who enjoys salads, try to top one with roasted beets and Brussels sprouts, cheese, nuts, blueberries, and a vinaigrette with olive oil within it. You can then serve it with a steak, salmon, sardines, turkey, or whatever your protein of choice is. By eating this salad rather than simple lettuce and Ranch salad you will receive many more benefits, nutrients, and remain satisfied. Of course, if you don't care for a salad, there are many other options of healthy dishes you can enjoy with a wide-range of nutrient-rich vegetables.

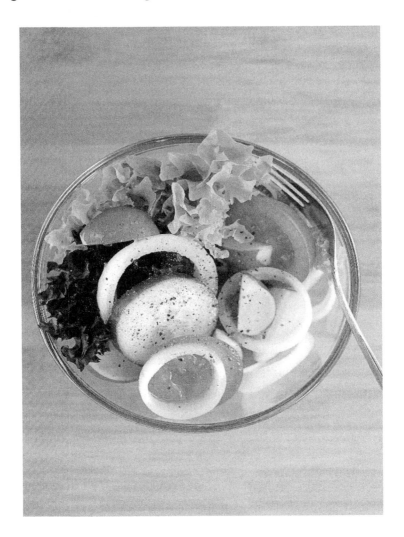

Fruits

Eating fruits like grapes and melons will be refreshing during your eating window and allow you to have some natural sugars originating from within the fruits so that you can still maintain your healthy diet. Because these fruits tend to have high water content, they'll be helping you stay hydrated too. If you are someone with a sweet tooth, it can be helpful to replace sweets with moderate amounts of these refreshing fruits. Before long, you can find that rather than craving cake you crave a cold slice of watermelon.

Fiber-rich fruits such as apples and pears can be a wonderful addition, as well. These fruits can be surprisingly filling, especially when served with protein such as some sliced chicken or nut butter to dip them in. If you want a real treat, you can always sauté an apple or pear with some coconut oil and cinnamon before topping it with some creamy almond butter. You will be full, satisfied, and enjoy a wide range of phytonutrients. Although, be sure to eat these fruits with the peel intact, as the peel is what contains a majority of the phytonutrients you require. If you remove the peel, you also remove most of the health-promoting qualities.

Avocados are the highest calorie fruit so it might seem counter-intuitive to eat them when you're trying to lose weight. Yet, the high content of monosaturated fat is extremely filling. Studies have found that having just half an avocado for breakfast can keep you full for much longer into the day. If that weren't a good enough reason to enjoy avocados, they are also high in many vitamins and minerals such as vitamin K, potassium, vitamin C, folate, vitamin E, and more. They have even been found to increase heart health, lower the risk of developing cancer, decrease the risk of metabolic syndrome, boost weight loss, prevent insulin resistance, and the list only goes on. Get some Avocados into your life!

Fruit Type	Carbs	Serving Size
Peach	7.26	¾
Plum plums	10.02	1 ½
Tomato	2.69	1 small vine tomato
Blueberry	12.09	¾ cup
Blackberry	4.31	¾ cup
Raspberry	5.44	¾ cup
Strawberry	5.68	¾ cup
Cranberry whole	8.37	1 c.
Melon honeydew balls	5.68	8
Cantaloupe (cantaloupe balls)	7.26	7
Watermelon (watermelon balls)	7.15	8
Coconut	6.23	1 cup
Lemon	6	one-half

Nuts and Seeds

If you have some time during your eating window, try snacking on healthy nuts like cashews, peanuts, pistachios, or almonds. There are so many to choose from, and you can easily incorporate them by tossing them into a salad or even in the main dish. They are packed with vitamins and minerals, contain healthy fats which increase only your "good" cholesterol level, and they're even a great source of protein However, be sure that you're choosing to eat raw nuts or dry roasted nuts. When nuts are covered in chocolate or sugar, then you're losing the health benefits. Pumpkin seeds are a great source of fat and fiber which can help you feel full for longer. They also contain magnesium, zinc, and manganese which give you energy

Chia seeds can easily be added into a variety of dishes, as they are tiny and lack much flavor. Despite this, they can be delicious when added to liquids since they create a gel, which can even be used to create a healthy pudding These micro-sized seeds contain protein, fiber, and healthy fats. Along with those nutrients, they contain micronutrients, which are the vitamins and minerals our bodies require. Some of these that are within chia seeds include zinc, magnesium, calcium, potassium, manganese, phosphorous, thiamine, niacin, and vitamin B12.

Sesame seeds are another tiny seed that packs a punch. But, unlike chia seeds, sesame seeds are known for their flavor. When ground into butter sesame is known as tahini, which is commonly added to hummus. But sesame seeds can also be used within sauces, as a topping, and even to crust meat before pan-frying it. Sesame seeds are high in phytonutrients, vitamin E, and vitamin K. They have been shown to lower stress, improve blood pressure, manage depression, increase skin health, reduce anemia, boost oral hygiene, lower stress, and manage the symptoms of rheumatoid arthritis.

You should keep nuts in moderation. Otherwise, they may cause weight gain, but it is advisable to eat a serving a day. A single serving of nuts is usually about an average handful. Almonds are a wonderful source of nut which can increase weight loss, improve heart health, boost energy, lower your risk of developing cancer, and prevent gallstones from developing.

Fats

People may recommend against eating fat, because of the calories it contains. But it is a misconception that fat makes you fat. Instead, the fat you consume will help your body stay satisfied during a long fast and will be used to create ketones, one of the healthiest sources of fuel for the human body. For this reason, it's important to consume a moderate number of healthy fats. Of course, if you are pairing intermittent fasting with the ketogenic diet, you will consume a higher number of fats while eating a lower number of carbohydrates.

One of the best sources of fats you can choose is coconut oil. This is because coconut is the highest fat with medium-chain triglycerides. This is great because these fat molecules, often simply referred to as MCTs, are able to be digested much more quickly than other fats. Due to this, you can gain energy more quickly. The liver can also easily transmute MCTs into ketones, which is especially helpful to keep you satisfied and energized during a fast. Along with these benefits, coconut oil has been shown to lower cholesterol, improve heart health, boost brain function, and more.

Olive oil is another excellent oil choice. The healthy fats within olives and their oil have been shown to improve heart health, lower cholesterol, increase brain health, boost weight loss, decrease the risk of cancer, strengthen bones, and more. When choosing olive oil try to find extra virgin olive oil to attain the benefits from the phytonutrients.

One of the tastiest fat options is grass-fed butter. Just as grass-fed meat is superior to grain-fed meat, the same is true of the butter. This is because grass-fed butter is much higher in nutrients and healthy fats. You may be worried about the saturated fats within butter, but it is a type of saturated fat with health-promoting qualities. Grass-fed butter has been shown to lower bad cholesterol and raise good cholesterol, greatly improving cardiovascular health in the process. If you are looking for grass-fed butter, it's best to get it locally, but if you are unable to most grocery stores sell Kerrygold, which is a delicious grass-fed Irish butter.

Tea

Drinking green tea during your fasts is a great habit to get into. This is because it contains caffeine to help you feel full, but it also contains something called thymine which keeps you mentally alert and focused without the jittery side effects coffee can bring. Also, it's been proven to help burn more belly fat.

Chapter 8:

Tips & Tricks to Help You Succeed

If you're thinking of getting started on an intermittent fasting schedule, we have some tips and tricks to help you succeed. The first 5 days will be the hardest, as you feel frequent hunger pangs and are going to be tempted by what you can't have. But, once you begin to adjust your day to your fasting routine, you will notice the time flies faster. Not only that, but your body will become adjusted and naturally feel less hungry during the fasting periods.

First Do Your Research

Just as you're reading this book to learn more about intermittent fasting, it's important that you're first aware of what fasting requires and all the pros and cons. Before making any changes to your diet, you should talk to your doctor to ensure that you are not underweight or jeopardizing your health if you are on any medication or have an illness. I've mentioned this several times throughout the book because it's extremely important and most people still don't do it!

Define Your Motivation

Remind yourself why you are going to these lengths and devoting yourself to a fasting routine. Are you trying to lose weight? Do you want to lower your cholesterol? Do you want to avoid snacking throughout the day and raising your blood sugar since diabetes runs in your family? Motivate yourself with whatever your goal is, so you are better focused and see the end goal of a skipping meal or two today.

Don't be Ashamed of Starting Slowly

Fasting is a tough habit to get into, and there's no shame in admitting that you are having a hard time completing your fasting window. Don't just jump into a 16 hour fast. Instead, work your way there slowly by cutting out snacks from your diet and skipping a meal or two. Train yourself by not having any snacks in the house and eating just one or two filling meals a day. Keep yourself hydrated and drink tea or coffee to get you through the day. The more you do it the easier it becomes.

Keep Yourself Busy

Think of it this way, the busier you are, the less time you'll have to focus on your growling stomach. One of the best ways to avoid thinking about food is to ensure you have enough to do during the day. Filling your time with work, family time, reading, exercising, crafting, volunteering, or whatever allows you to have a busy day so that you don't even realize that lunchtime is over. It makes your fasting time go much faster if you keep yourself occupied.

Avoid Temptations

This can be a bit hard to do if you're fasting during the day or have business lunches but remind yourself of your end goal and don't put yourself in a situation where you might be tempted. Even if you're out to eat with a bunch of friends and tell yourself you will only have water or coffee, you might be tempted to just try "one" thing, and you'll have broken your fast. So, try and stay away from food-related gatherings or convening at restaurants or bars during your fasting hours. Instead, choose a neutral location your friends can still enjoy and where you won't feel tempted. Then, you can, later on, enjoy going to food-centered locations when you aren't in the middle of a fast. For instance, if you have just finished a fast, you may choose to go out to eat with friends. You can break your fast with a large healthy meal at a restaurant you truly enjoy. But, make sure that the food you choose will sustain you. It is better to eat a steak with a sweet potato and broccoli rather than a large slice of cheesecake.

Stay Hydrated

We've said it time and time again, but water is key so that you are not at risk of becoming dehydrated. Drinking enough water is another way to "fool" your body into feeling sated. You'll feel less irritable too. Be sure to increase your daily water intake. Keep a reusable water bottle with you in reach so you can take a few sips as you're working. If you're fasting, you should have at least half your body mass in ounces of water. This means that if you weight one-hundred and fifty pounds you should be drinking a minimum of seventy-five ounces in water. It seems like a lot, but as long as you are keeping your water bottle handy and refiling it, you'll be surprised how fast you reach your goal.

Include Caffeine in Your Routine

You may not be an avid coffee or tea drinker now, but you want to get into the habit of it when you are fasting. Caffeine has been proven to dull your appetite which means it'll allow your stomach to feel like it's being filled with food even if all you're having is a cup of coffee. Be sure you're not using cream or sugar though.

Those are extra calories that will add up over time. Next time when you're delaying breakfast or feeling a craving after dinner, try having a cup of coffee or night time tea instead. You can even try calorie-free gum which can keep you occupied until your cravings pass.

Don't Fast in Stressful Situations

Situations of grief or potential health emergencies can be terrible, and cause stress on your body. Don't force yourself to fast during such emergencies if they occur within your life, because you may only be doing your body harm. Sometimes with situations like that, you need to sit down and have a comforting meal. Coffee and tea will not do the trick. But just because you aren't fasting don't allow yourself to binge eat. You can tell yourself that you'll let yourself enjoy a comforting meal, but remind yourself that it won't solve your problems, it's not a solution, and that you can't go back for seconds. Rather than eating an entire tub of ice cream, you may allow yourself a single ice cream cone.

Use a Buddy to Keep You Motivated

By tackling intermittent fasting together with a friend, you will find yourself much more motivated and encouraged. This will give you a person to go to the gym with, relax within a safe environment without food, and know that you won't be constantly pushed to try and eat something or order something off the menu. If you have a friend who is also interested in intermittent fasting and gaining the health benefits, try spending time together while fasting and motivating each other.

Get a Good Night's Sleep

Sleep is important for health in general, but it's especially going to be important when you are doing intermittent fasting. Why? Well, because when you're asleep, you can't realize you're hungry. Be sure to set up your sleep time so it aligns with some of your fasting windows so you can spend a chunk of it asleep. That means if you're fasting after dinner until late morning, be sure to go to bed early so you can avoid temptation and still feel like you've fallen asleep on a full stomach. Have water or tea before bed to keep you feeling full, and ensure you're having some restful sleep, so you don't wake up cranky the next day.

Another reason that sleep is important is that when you lack sleep your hormones become unbalanced. The stress hormone cortisol increases, which causes your weight loss to stall and increases the feeling that you need to eat. Similarly, the hormones ghrelin and leptin which also control hunger signals and satiety become unbalanced, leading you to eat more calories than you otherwise would. If you sleep well regularly, you will find that you have much more success with both fasting and weight loss.

Season Your Food with Herbs and Spices

I'm a big fan of spicy food. It may sound like a little thing but adding some extra herbs and seasoning over your meals when you're eating them can actually help you feel full longer. It wakes up your taste buds, and ingredients such as garlic, spices, and vinegar contain a non-significant number of calories so you can still maintain a healthy diet.

By flavoring your food more, you can also increase your satisfaction. Rather than eating a bland chicken breast, you can enjoy a full-flavored meal that keeps you happy. You won't feel

100

the need to break your fast because you truly enjoy the food you make.

Toss out the Junk Food

The more temptations you have around, the more you want to snack when you shouldn't. To avoid this, be sure you've cleaned out your pantry and fridge and that you have gotten rid of snacks and junk food, so you don't stumble upon some cookies or chips. Instead, focus on stocking your kitchen with healthy ingredients you can use to make energy-rich, healthy, and delicious meals.

Monitor Your Progress

This doesn't mean you should obsess over your weight or get frustrated if your weight loss isn't going as fast as you thought it would. But, weigh yourself at the end of every week or 2 weeks so you can see the numbers on the scale and how much weight you've lost. Whether it's 4 pounds or 1 pound, or half a pound, use the free online apps or keep a chart and motivate yourself that you're reaching your goal.

Along with weighing yourself, you should also measure yourself. This is because muscle weighs more than fat, so even if the scale isn't moving you may be losing fat and inches. This often occurs when the scale stays stagnant, but you still go down a pant size. Failing that a good indicator of your fat % is simply by observing how your clothes fit on you.

Workout Slowly

You don't want to push yourself into training or high-intensity exercises when you first begin fasting. Instead, allow yourself to get into a routine of some exercise to further encourage your body to lose weight. Whether you begin lightly with yoga, Pilates, or a walk around the block, and then work your way up to the treadmill. This is a start that will help you feel energized and gain the benefits of exercise.

Meditate

If you are feeling anxious or frazzled during your day, you might be tempted to break your fast. Instead, take some time and use relaxation techniques to combat your negative thoughts. Try some meditation strategies, listen to white noise or calming music, try yoga or breathing exercises to help you feel relaxed again. Motivate yourself that you've made it this far through your fasting window and that you can complete the rest

Keep an Eye Out for Discomfort

The most important factor first and foremost is your health. If for some reason you feel any discomfort, whether it's nausea, stomach pains, muscle cramps, or dizziness and fatigue, it's okay for you to break your fast and put your health first. It could be your blood sugar is too low, or maybe you haven't had enough to drink today. You know your body best, so it's important that you put your comfort first.

Chapter 9:

Pairing the Ketogenic Diet with Intermittent Fasting for Success

The ketogenic diet is perfect when paired with intermittent fasting. While fasting is not required when you are on the ketogenic diet, and vice versa, the two systems greatly benefit one another, and I have enjoyed massive benefits from combining the two. But first, what is the ketogenic diet? In this chapter, we will answer the basics of the ketogenic diet and how you can pair it with intermittent fasting for optimal success.

While you may be unsure what the ketogenic diet entails, you have most likely heard of the term 'keto.' This is because the ketogenic diet is often simply shortened to keto, as it has become increasingly well-known and popular. While the diet has been around for nearly a century for the treatment in epilepsy, it has only recently become popular to a wider audience due to its ability to increase sustainable weight loss while allowing a person to enjoy a wide range of healthy foods and remain sated.

The ketogenic diet was first created after the previously mentioned studies on fasting for the treatment of epilepsy. Not long after intermittent fasting was found to be successful, researchers found that a diet low in carbohydrates with a moderate amount of protein and high amount of fats can be sustained while maintaining the same beneficial aspects as fasting.

This is largely because when you are in a fasted state, your body will create ketones in order to fuel itself and increase production of mitochondrial cells. When you are on an extremely low-carbohydrate diet, your body goes into the same process of creating ketones, in order to fuel the portions of your brain that are unable to be fueled by fat. Because the ketogenic diet and intermittent fasting have many of the same beneficial effects upon your body, you can simply combine the two to reach even greater success and further benefits. If you use the ketogenic diet while fasting, you will find that you are sated and energized for longer periods of time. If you add intermittent fasting in while on the ketogenic diet, you can experience further healing and weight loss benefits than with the keto lifestyle alone. The two together work as a beautiful harmony and melody. On their own, they may be beautiful, but together they can be amazing.

While you are eating on the ketogenic diet all grains, legumes, beans, high-sugar fruits, and starchy vegetables will be removed from your diet. Don't get me wrong; these ingredients do have their benefits. You can attain the nutrition your body requires if you eat healthy low-carb ingredients in their place. This doesn't mean you will completely forsake eating carbohydrates, but you will simply choose ingredients that contain a lower amount.

While you are trying to control your carbohydrate intake, you will need to be familiar with net carbohydrates. Total carbohydrates are the number of complete carbs within an ingredient or meal. For instance, an average apple contains twenty-five total carbohydrates. Apples and other foods also contain fiber. This fiber is not digested by your body. Instead, it is used to benefit your digestion and nutrient absorption before being expelled. Because of this, you don't count carbohydrates deriving from the fiber in the net carbohydrate count. Let's look at an apple again. While an apple may contain twenty-five total carbs, it also contains four grams of fiber. Therefore, after removing the fiber count from the total carbohydrate count, you are left with a net carb count of twenty-one grams.

However, apples are generally too high in carbohydrates to be consumed on a regular basis on the ketogenic diet. This is due to their natural sugar content. Instead, you want to choose ingredients that are lower. Strawberries are a wonderful choice because an entire serving only contains eight net carbohydrates. But, how do you know how many carbohydrates you can enjoy? Carbs, along with protein and fat are what are known as macronutrients. These are the nutrients that you require in the largest proportion. In order to know how much you need in each category of macronutrients, you can find many keto macro calculators online. At the end of this book, in the resources section, you can find several macro calculators which are great. But, put simply, your macros are determined by your weight, activity level, gender, and weight loss goals. This will look different for every person, but in general, you will consume between twenty-five and thirty net carbs during the course of a day.

Along with the net carbohydrates, you will be consuming a moderate amount of protein. The exact amount varies on your weight and activity level, but in general, you will need twenty to thirty percent of your day's calories to originate from protein. This is vital because if you don't eat enough protein, your immune system will weaken, your muscles will begin to atrophy, and you will be at a higher risk of developing diseases. Thankfully, it is not that difficult to include your day's recommended protein if you enjoy plenty of meat, fish, seafood, cheese, nuts, and eggs.

The ketogenic diet is primarily made up of fats. This is because after you consume your required protein level and attain twenty-five net carbohydrates, you will need the remainder of your day's calorie goal to source from something else. The remaining option is fat. Therefore, it's important that you source healthy types of fat. You want to avoid unhealthy processed fats such as corn, peanut, and soy oil. Instead, choose whole or the oil of avocados and olives, coconut oil, nuts, seeds, lard, fatty meats, and grass-fed butter. These sources of fat are full of health-promoting properties that studies have shown time and again treat and prevent disease.

The ketogenic diet may be different from what you are used to, but when paired with intermittent fasting it is a powerful process. When your body is low on glucose and begins to create ketones as a fuel source you are in a state of ketosis. This state is most often reached due to the ketogenic diet and fasting. Whatever your reason for choosing to begin a keto and fasting lifestyle, you can experience many benefits. Brain health is especially impacted by these processes, which is why they are often used in the treatment of epilepsy and Alzheimer's disease. This is because many neurological diseases share a commonality in being deficient in the way they process fuel for energy.

While the cells in the brain consume quite a bit of energy just to survive, many diseases prevent these cells from consuming their very life source. Thankfully, both ketones and fat are a much more effective and efficient energy source for the brain than glucose from carbs. This will enable the cells to more easily absorb their nutrients and take a slight burden off of them. Imagine, if an engine is constantly running it will break down more easily. However, if you give an engine breaks to cool off and recover along with a better fuel source it can long outlive its competition.

Speaking of better fuel, the ketogenic diet allows the brain to have a larger supply of healthy fats. These fats, in turn, decrease inflammation both in the brain and throughout the remainder of the human body. By decreasing the inflammation levels, you are able to experience less pain, be at a lower risk of developing a disease, and possibly even treat chronic illnesses.

There are various types of the ketogenic diet, which is important to be aware of for people on various lifestyles. The numbers we have given for protein and carbohydrates have both been for the standard ketogenic diet. At the name suggests, this is the go-to keto lifestyle which fits most people and easy to manage. This is ideal for people who only exercise occasionally and who don't practice high-intensity exercises such as bodybuilding, HIIT, and CrossFit. The number of calories you eat on the standard ketogenic diet, and all of them for that matter, will vary based on your body weight, activity level, and weight goals. For instance, a bodybuilder will require more calories than someone who is not physically active.

Along with the standard ketogenic diet you may be interested in the targeted ketogenic diet. This form of the diet is ideal for people who practice bodybuilding, HIIT, CrossFit, and other high-intensity exercises. This form of keto is especially helpful for people who are only just beginning high-intensity exercises or who practice them irregularly because it allows them to burn off the extra glucose and retain a state of ketosis.

With the targeted ketogenic diet, you simply increase your carb count on exercise days. Thirty minutes prior to a high-intensity workout you can consume an added twenty-five to thirty net carbohydrates from a healthy source. Some great choices are fruits, beets, sweet potatoes, and whole grains. By doing this, your body will process the carbs before your workout and refuel your muscles with ATP energy.

Remember, this is only needed for high-intensity workouts. You can perform aerobics and cardio perfectly fine on the standard ketogenic diet because they do not rely on ATP energy.

The cyclical ketogenic diet is for people who workout at high-intensities four or more times a week every week. This is because the cyclical ketogenic diet consists of loading up on carbs for a few days before continuing with the standard ketogenic diet. This allows a person to have quite a bit of ATP energy for their workout, but it is harder to schedule. You also have to be careful to stick to the feeding and workout schedule strictly. Otherwise, you will be unable to maintain ketosis. For this reason, we tend to prefer the targeted ketogenic diet for high-intensity workouts rather than the cyclical ketogenic diet.

Lastly is the high protein ketogenic diet, which bodybuilders frequently utilize. Carbohydrates are not necessary in order to gain muscle mass. Instead, protein is much more significant toward reaching a goal of muscle building than carbs. While some bodybuilders may choose to carb up for a boost, this only increases their efficiency by one to two percent. You would be better off focusing on protein, the ketogenic diet, and intermittent fasting than eating carbs.

The high protein ketogenic diet was created with this in mind. In order to help those people gain muscle mass, it is generally recommended to consume one gram of protein for each pound of body weight on this diet. This means before consuming carbs or fat a bodybuilder's first concern on the high-protein ketogenic diet should be protein. It doesn't matter if the protein comes from eggs, meat, fish, or cheese.

If they are hoping to put on more weight, it's recommended to consume an increase of two-hundred and fifty to five-hundred calories higher than your standard caloric intake. Remember, if you are taking up bodybuilding you will gain more muscle in the beginning and will find the most benefit. After you have been bodybuilding for a time you will gradually begin to experience a slower and more manageable muscle increase. Therefore, you will require a smaller calorie surplus.

You may be wondering what you can and can't eat on the ketogenic diet. Put simply; you can enjoy meats, fish, high-fat cheeses, low-starch vegetables, berries, nuts, and seeds. Be sure to check the labels of foods you are eating so that you don't exceed twenty-five net carbs during the course of a day. You should even check the vegetables you eat, which you can easily track in many nutrition and diet smartphone apps. But, let's go over a few of the ingredients you shouldn't eat in order to clear up any questions you might have on the subject:

Grains

Yes, grains are healthy and full of fiber. They contain quite a high number of net carbs, making them incompatible with the standard ketogenic diet. Of course, if you are using the targeted ketogenic diet, you may enjoy a very small serving directly prior to a workout, and on the cyclical keto diet, you may enjoy some on carb load days. Otherwise, you should completely avoid all grains.

Many Fruits

You can enjoy berries to a great extent, avocados, olives, lemons, limes, and even melon in moderation from time to time. You should focus on low-starch vegetables in order to get many of your nutrients instead of fruit. While fruit, like grains, is healthy, it contains quite a number of natural sugars. These sugars will cause blood sugar and insulin reactions, which is something you want to avoid.

Starchy Vegetables

Yes, potatoes are a vegetable. But, while they have healthy aspects, you are much better off eating low-starch vegetables such as kale, cruciferous vegetables, bell peppers, and others. This is because starchy vegetables, such as potatoes, are high in carbs. A single medium potato contains forty-three net carbs, a sweet potato contains twenty-three net carbs, and a half cup of corn contains fifty-five net carbs These are all high on the glycemic index, causing it to raise your blood sugar and insulin. Once the blood sugar crash, you will experience increased hunger and cravings, causing you to be more likely to overeat. Plus, these foods are so high in carbohydrates that they will prevent you from attaining ketosis.

If you are someone who loves potatoes, you can often find recipes replacing them with turnips, daikon radishes, kohlrabi, rutabaga, celery root, and cauliflower. I know, it may be different, but don't knock it until you've tried it.

Low-Fat Dairy

You can enjoy low-carb high-fat dairies such as cheeses, cream cheese, and heavy cream on the ketogenic diet. However, you should avoid all milk and low-carb options such as low-fat cheese. This is because the dairy options that are made to be low in fat are naturally higher in carbohydrates, which you want to avoid.

Cashews, Pistachios, and Chestnuts

You are able to enjoy nuts and seeds on the ketogenic diet in moderation. However, there are exceptions. Certain nuts, specifically cashews, pistachios, and chestnuts, are simply too high in net carbs to be justified. For instance, a single small serving of cashews contains nine net carbohydrates while not even having a full gram of fiber to offer. For this reason, it is best to enjoy almonds, walnuts, pecans, macadamia, and other nuts instead.

Natural "Healthy" Sweeteners

You can enjoy most sugar alcohols on the ketogenic diet. This is because erythritol and xylitol are not processed by the body as sugar but are instead dumped along with the fiber you eat.

However, other natural sweeteners such as honey, agave, maple, and dates should be avoided completely. These may be seen as a superior lower glycemic option, but the truth is that they are all high in carbs and cause a spike in blood sugar and insulin. If you want something sweet, instead reach for erythritol, stevia, or even monk fruit extract.

Alcohol

Not all alcohol may be high in carbohydrates, such as vodka and rum. But, many types of alcohol are high in carbs. Although, this is not the only reason you should avoid alcohol when you are on the ketogenic diet and intermittent fasting. The main reason is that alcohol interferes with the creation of ketones and weight loss, this then prevents you from being able to reach the very goal you began your new lifestyle for. While your body is attempting to burn off the alcohol, it will be unable to process any calories you have eaten or attempt weight loss. It's also important to know that when you are in a state of ketosis you can get drunk and hangovers more easily.

Chapter 10:

IF and me

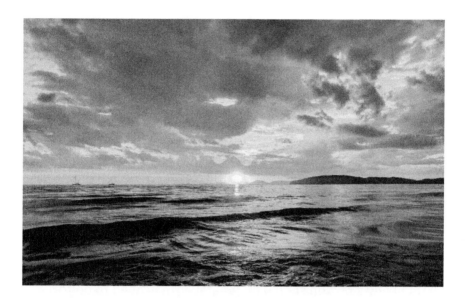

In this chapter I would like to share more of my own personal fitness journey with you in the hope that it gives you some ideas which you could perhaps use for yourself. This chapter is not strictly IF related as it's more about my general personal experiences with eating and fitness during times when I'm not following an eating method or, particular diet. In other words, my normal or usual routine. If perhaps you aren't particularly interested, then please feel free to skip to the next chapter.

These day's I use different tools and methods to keep lean and fit, depending on my needs and how I feel at the time. I now have a healthy relationship with food and alcohol, and I attribute this to me not denying myself of the things that I really enjoy. Moderation as always is definitely key here.

As I've said before, Intermittent Fasting is an extremely effective method of fat loss. These days I can dip in and out of this method of eating depending on what my current goals are. We are only human and even with the greatest of intentions life often gets in the way. As John Lennon said, 'Life is what happens while you're busy making other plans'. You may fall off the wagon, have a night out with your friends, attend events, weddings BBQ's or whatever and deviate from you diet or eating plan. That's fine so long as you have the discipline to get back on track however that's where some people give up and go back to their old ways. You need to be persistent and determined to win this struggle.

Our bodies are in a constant change and at any given time I might want to lose some bodyfat or gain muscle mass. I am now at a stage where I can use and benefit from either IF or the Keto, Vegan or the Mediterranean diet at any time. I can pick and choose depending on what I feel like doing and eating. I believe that initially a person should do whatever they need to do to reach their target fitness and if your chosen diet or eating plan is palatable and manageable long term then absolutely stick to it. However, we need to live too. We should enjoy the foods we love. The feelgood benefits of a little of what you love every now and then is worth the calories provided we don't overdo it and get back on track. I mean, what's the point in being lean but miserable? I personally want to sample many different types of food and drink and I want to eat chocolate or drink alcohol when I please. As I said I'm not an extremist, I'm an average guy who wants to enjoy life to the full and also keep fit and healthy. I basically want my cake and to eat it.

I would love to share some other small health tips that are perhaps a little unconventional but that I've found to be very effective for me. I have successfully managed to naturally bust stress, depression and insomnia and trimmed body fat and gained lean muscle at the same time by consistently practicing some little habits and rituals. These little habits are easy to follow and have served me very well they are easy to maintain long term.

In my experience, once you get to your target weight you can then practically eat and drink whatever you want if you control your portion sizes.

I love to experiment with food and health supplements. In my workplace they'll say, "What's he doing now?" as I mix various weird and wonderful healthy concoctions. These have generally worked out very well for me over the years. Below are some examples of some methods and habits that have certainly helped me in my quest to be as fit as possible without being too obsessed with strict dieting etc.

I've observed that the main reason most people fail to lose bodyfat and get fit is because they don't stick to a routine that works for them long term. After around 2 months of 'healthy eating' they get bored and go back to their old habits. They also are not 100% honest with themselves about what they eat and drink.

Yoyo diets rarely work. Fad diets and mega strict health regimes are often too hard to stick to long term and I like I said I still want to enjoy wine, beer, curries and chips and chocolate or whatever else I fancy, whenever I chose and yet still have a decent physique with low bodyfat and some muscle definition. You'll see in the photo of me below that I am no model! I'm not particularly muscle bound, and I perhaps don't have a perfect looking torso but that's the point really. I don't try to be perfect. I'm just an average guy in his mi- forties who wants to enjoy being quite fit while enjoying eating and drinking whatever I please within reason.

With some little healthy habits here and there, I'm living proof that this can be achievable. The main ingredient for success has been a strong will power and determination. If you truly want something, and I mean REALLY want something you will move mountains to get it. You'll be like a kind of super determined Terminator who will not stop until you get what you want.

It's that sort of mindset that you should adopt to laser focus your mind into making massive changes be it for your health or career or whatever else. I'll add that it gets easier to find that focus once you start to make small changes to feel more positive and healthier in yourself. Feeling positive has several knock-on effects. Once you start to sleep better and deal with nagging pain or anxiety, your positivity will return with a vengeance.

Now I'm not suggesting to you that you do what I do but have a look anyway. This is my current usual eating routine. It's not a diet as such it's just a routine that I can use now that I am comfortable with my weight.

- Drink approximately 1 pint of water (ideally with the juice of a lemon) in the morning before eating or drinking anything. Drink water throughout the day, even if it makes you urinate more frequently.

- Always eat breakfast. My favorite is porridge oats, whole milk, peanut butter, honey, chia seeds, desiccated

116

coconut, flaxseed, blueberries/raspberries and cinnamon. This lot takes less than 4 minutes to make. It's a powerhouse of nutrients and the cinnamon aide's fat loss and lowers blood pressure. You could even add a little chili pepper! Yes, chili pepper! It will ramp up your metabolism and is a great anti-inflammatory. It tastes good too.

- Snack throughout the day with half an avocado, a banana or a handful of unsalted unroasted nuts or full fat natural yogurt which you can add fruit to. I like to add macca powder to mine to help maintain healthy testosterone levels.

- Limit your coffee to 1-2 cups per day.

- Drink green tea. Take omega 3, 6 fish oils during the day. Take ZMA vitamins before bed (Magnesium, Zinc and B6)

- Just now I take 6 drops of 5% CBD oil by tincture orally, placed under my tongue.

- Mix a small amount of apple cider vinegar with coconut oil and the juice of a lemon. Add hot water and a dash of cayenne pepper. This little concoction really helps burn bodyfat and balances your hormones. Seriously.

- Only eat crisps/cakes or biscuits very occasionally as a treat. Same with chocolate. I eat plain chocolate in moderation. The less you eat of these types of foods the less you crave them. The more you eat them the more you want them.

- Try to eat at least some veggies and protein every single day. Cut back a little bit on fast carbs like white bread and pasta. Try having brown bread and whole wheat pasta instead. Eat as much oily fish as you can. I eat tuna and salmon a lot. I also eat well over the recommended amount of eggs. In fact, I drink raw eggs every other day! You should certainly not try this. This goes against every health article or guidance I've ever read however I have been doing this for over 20 years without issue. I only drink free range eggs. Why do I do this? Because for me it's the ultimate convenient protein shake and while it's not particularly easy to drink I do get real benefits from it. I know it sounds a bit disgusting and I guess maybe it is. I blame it on the Rocky films I watched as a kid. Again, I do not advise you to do this. I am simply telling you what honestly works for me. It might not work for you and you could end up very ill if you try it. You are much safer eating more cooked eggs perhaps in an omelet or hard boiled.

- This sounds obvious but don't eat unless you are hungry. There's nothing wrong with going without food until you are feeling hungry. Likewise, you don't need to eat everything and leave the plate squeaky clean if you don't want to. Eat until your satisfied and leave the rest if you don't need it. If you know you ate too much over a weekend or a holiday or whatever then reign it back in a little over the next few days. Some people don't seem to know when they've had enough, and they seem to almost 'inhale' large amounts of food each day.

- Walk each day. Or at least move around quite a bit. Don't sit still at a desk all day. Try to exercise in some form or other around 2-3 times a week and integrate it into your lifestyle. Find an activity you really enjoy like cycling, running, swimming, dancing, weights training etc. and make it your habit to do it throughout your life. Do it because you enjoy doing it not because you're 'exercising'. No matter what age you are you should consider doing resistance training i.e. weights training. There are huge

118

benefits to be had here including better sleep, which improves mood, which lessens anxiety, which promotes positivity...you see where I'm going here? Add CBD oil to this little mix and I promise you'll experience big positive changes over time.

- Drink wine or whatever you fancy in moderation. If you do have a heavy drinking session, then drink water throughout the night and drink 2 pints of water before bed and you'll have less of a hangover the next day since a hangover is basically caused by dehydration. I'll admit I love red wine. Perhaps a little too much. I'm very rarely drunk as such, but I do drink a little wine every weekend because I enjoy it. I told you that I was a Scotsman, didn't I? I do occasionally stop drinking for weeks and months at a time and when I do I see improvements on how I look and feel. Again, moderation is key. Do what you enjoy but do it sensibly and don't do anything too much. Be honest with yourself about exactly what you eat and drink.

A bit more on exercise.

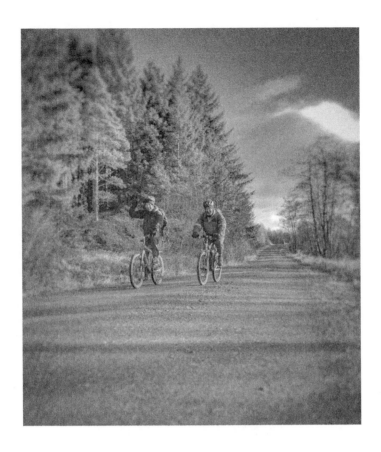

I would like to say to anyone who is suffering from mild to medium stress/anxiety/depression/insomnia that simple exercise can work wonders for you. Cycling, walking or jogging, playing football or gardening are all great examples.

Fresh air and an elevated heart rate are powerful natural anti-depressants. Exercise will produce endorphins and can make you feel on top of the world. High intensity exercise can make you feel like a bit of a superhero. A perfect combination would be outdoor exercise at the weekends and weights training during the week. All subject to your goals and what you want to achieve of course, be it fat loss or muscle gain or both.

Even simple little changes will all add up over time. Walking to the shops or strolling around the block at lunch time can really make a difference. It doesn't necessarily need to be high intensity, especially not at the start. Often making the initial decision to make a major change can seem like the daunting bit to some people. Be bold and be brave. Tell yourself that you're gonna do this. If you sometimes work in an office block like I do, then try taking the stairs rather than the lift. Even start by taking the stairs down at first then attempt to climb up them in the morning. Again, it all adds up.

If you work on the 3rd floor and each floor has two flights of 9 steps you will burn around 4200 calories per year by just taking the stairs. Or around 6300 calories if you're on the 4th floor. 8300 on the 5th floor and 10400 on the 6th! That's quite a lot don't you think? You will lose fat doing this. My favorite exercise of all time however is cycling.

I just love how off-road cycling makes me feel. It's perfect interval training and zooming down hills is exciting. It's a bit like being a kid again. When you are cycling in the countryside either by yourself or with friends you can experience a physical and spiritual uplift that is very powerful on your mind and body. It can destroy stress or at least make it much more manageable. It will help you sleep better and vastly improve your mood. You might consider giving cycling a try for yourself.

Remember that fitness and wellbeing is 80% nutrition. Get your own nutrition and exercise sorted out and I promise you that you will sleep better and naturally reduce anxiety and depression and you will feel mentality and physically supercharged.

The benefits of exercise cannot be overemphasized. Another interesting discovery of mine has been CBD Hemp Oil. It has helped me because it has made me feel calm and helped me sleep

121

which has aided my recovery after exercise. Faster recovery means getting fitter quicker. You could say that the benefits I've experienced from CBD have had a knock-on effect on other areas.

Years of training in Bruce Lees brutal martial art Jeet Kune Do while exhilarating at the time, left me with a couple of injuries which occasionally surface as a pain in my right wrist.

We had been training hard as always when I fractured my wrist on the hard floor of the large basement where we trained. It was a very painful experience and I almost let out a Bruce Lee like whoooaaaa! when it happened. CBD oil has helped me deal with this pain when it appears. Just taking my drops in my tincture has helped neutralize the pain along with performing its other little tasks like reducing my anxiety and helping me sleep etc. That's the cool thing about CBD oil. When you find the right brand and take the right dose it helps a few different things at once and it helps your body and mind to help naturally treat these ailments. CBD seems to just help it along which makes sense when you consider how our own ECS works.

We are all only human and stress present itself at any time which is quite normal. It's learning to recognize the signs and dealing with it before it gets out of hand which is very important. The right type of diet and exercise will help with this.

Oh, one more thing. If you have arthritis or joint inflammation another effective treatment which can be used out-with or alongside CBD oil and cream is something called Golden Paste. It contains Turmeric and Turmeric can work wonders on all sorts of ailments for you and your pets and I suggest you give it a try.

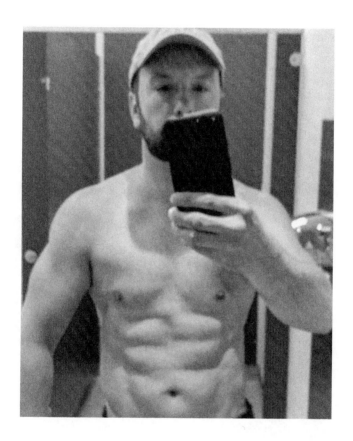

Here's me tensing up my abs in a rather flattering overhead light.
(I never, ever do sit ups or crunches.)

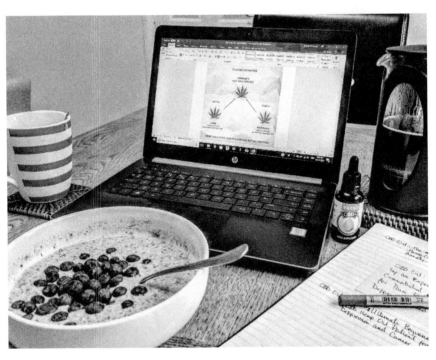

This is what my desk typically looked like while researching CBD Oil for another project. Note the super porridge, coffee and CBD tincture all within range.

Now CBD Oil is currently a hot topic and I have used it many times to help in my physical and mental training. It can help you keep calm and concentrate, which in turn can help in all areas of your life including following a new eating plan. Incidentally I am not an affiliate of CBD in any way whatsoever and I do not sell it. Again, I am simply and honestly telling you what works for me.

I felt it worthy of discussion since people are often confused about what CBD Oil is and what to look for when buying it. Below is a fictitious brand which I have made up however it will give you an idea of what to expect and what to look for should you wish to buy some online.

Browns Hemp Oil 1000mg-Organic CBD Hemp Oil for Pain and Stress Relief, Improved Mood, Better sleep, Skin Care (1000mg, 33.3mg per Serving x 30 Servings) $29.99

Product description

Browns CBD Hemp Oil Extract Supports:

- Omega 3 and Omega 6 Supplementation
- Rest and Relaxation*
- Anxiety Relief*
- Cortisol Manager*
- Quality Sleep Patterns*
- Inflammation and Joint Pain Relief*
- Nourishes Hair and Skin*
- Immune, Limbic, Neurogenic System Support*

* These statements have not been evaluated by the Food and Drug Administration. This product is not intended to diagnose, treat, cure, or prevent any disease.

Directions: Shake and squeeze 1-2 servings (1ml or 30 drops per 33.3mg serving) under tongue. Hold for 60 sec before swallowing. Use 1-3 times daily and consistently. Store cool.

Browns Blend:

Here at Browns Hemp Oil we are proud to use a full spectrum oil that includes the natural terpenes and antioxidants present in the hemp plant. Our products include all the phytonutrients present in the industrial hemp plant to give you the full effect of hemp oil. No artificial sweeteners, preservatives or pesticides.

Why buy Browns?

We're Scotland based and use only organically grown hemp from certified Scottish hemp farms. Our hemp is extracted through a state-of-the-art clean CO_2 process that leaves nutrients intact without using harmful solvents, and everything is tested for potency and safety.

Purchase with Confidence:

Our product is non-psychoactive with a THC content of 0.2%, and federally legal in all 50 states as it is derived from industrial hemp. We offer a full guarantee - if you are unhappy with any of our products, simply send it back within 30-days and we'll refund your order. Your statutory rights are unaffected.

Important information

Safety Information

Check with your doctor before ingesting any herbal supplements, consumption of herbal ingredients may cause allergies in certain individuals. If you have a known medical condition, you should consult with a healthcare professional before using this or any dietary supplement. If you have a history of allergies to herbal ingredients, do not consume this product. If pregnant, breastfeeding, or on a prescribed medication, consult your physician before use.

Legal Disclaimer

Browns Hemp Oil and these statements have not been evaluated by the Food and Drug Administration. This product is not intended to diagnose, treat, cure, or prevent any disease.

Statements regarding dietary supplements have not been evaluated by the FDA and are not intended to diagnose, treat, cure, or prevent any disease or health condition.

Ingredients

CBD 5% Hemp Seed Oil, Fractionated Coconut Oil, Peppermint Oil

Directions

Shake well and fill dropper with one 10mg serving (30 drops, about 1/2 of dropper). Squeeze drops underneath tongue and hold for 45 seconds before swallowing. Use 1-2 times daily. Store in a cool place out of sunlight.

Typical CBD Nutritional Value Label

Nutrition Facts

Serving Size 1 dropper (1mL)
Servings Per Container 15

Amount Per Serving	
Calories 7	Calories from Fat 7

	% Daily Values*
Total Fat 1g	2%
Saturated Fat 0g	0%
Trans Fat 0g	
Cholesterol 0mg	0%
Sodium 0mg	0%
Total Carbohydrate 0g	0%
Dietary Fiber 0g	0%
Sugars 0g	
Protein 0g	0%

*Percent Daily Values are based on a 2,000 calorie diet. Your Daily Values may be higher or lower depending on your calorie needs.

		Calories	2,000	2,500
Total Fat	Less than		65g	80g
Sat Fat	Less than		20g	25g
Cholesterol	Less than		300mg	300mg
Sodium	Less than		2400mg	2400mg
Total Carbohydrate			300g	375g
Dietary Fiber			25g	30g

For your information here's some bullet points on my CBD experience so far:

- Mixing 5 or 10% CBD oil with alcohol worked out fine for me with no real adverse effects. Mixing brands or methods of consumptions presented no issues.

- Combining 5 or 10% CBD oil with paracetamol, ibuprofen, co-codamol, antibiotics (amoxicillin) or cough mixtures was fine with no real adverse effects.

- Different brands with the exact same ingredients can still produce slightly different results. Some made me feel sleepy and some didn't. Some made me feel ever so slightly irritable on a moderate dose of 6 drops. The tincture pictured in this book is a 30 ml 5% CBD product from Holland and Barret and this brand makes me feel quite sleepy. It can relax me too however any more than 6 drops and I start feel very slightly irritated. Other brands with the same CBD content and carrier oil seemed to have less effects of any kind.

- Taking CBD on an empty stomach was ok. Effects were still felt within 20 minutes from a tincture.

- CBD didn't help my cold symptoms and it made no real difference to my mood or state of mind when I was sick. It won't help with a chest infection, cough or sore throat.

- It didn't show on a drug test and I never feel fuzzy or tired the next day unless I take the oil later as I've said. Driving or operating machinery isn't a problem for me at all.

- I'm not addicted to CBD. Stopping and starting again is easy and I don't believe that I've built up a tolerance to it. There are no noticeable withdrawal symptoms. There are no visible signs that you take CBD oil and I don't smell or sweat CBD oil smells. I don't need a loading phase with CBD oil like some say. The effects either work quite quickly that same day or don't work at all.

- 5 and 10% Tinctures have worked best for me. I don't mind using the tincture and the natural taste is not an issue for me. I usually take it orally under the tongue or occasionally I put it in food or I cook with it.

- I took one month's supply of 5% CBD in one evening and suffered no real side effects apart from a dry mouth and a slightly irritated feeling which made my skin feel just a little bit itchy. I also upset stomach the next morning probably due to taking 30ml of oil within a couple of hours. This gave me slight wind although I didn't feel uncomfortable. I slept very soundly that night and the next day I felt a little fuzzy for most of the morning. It cleared, and I felt fine. Over all taking too much CBD didn't cause any lasting harm that I could detect.

- Vapes and sprays didn't work as well as tinctures and capsules for me. Edibles are fine for variety although it can be tricky achieving a precise dosage per serving. CBD isn't cheap and the best value in my opinion comes from the tinctures and concentrates.

- CBD helps my anxiety and insomnia and my wrist pain. The natural feeling of calm helps with other areas like work and even relationships however the effects are not always consistent and sometimes it depends on my state of mind and current fitness levels. It is not always a miracle cure on its own with regards to a health tonic. It certainly lends a helping hand though.

- CBD seems to help balance my partners hormones around period time and it works well with evening primrose. Just a few drops of whatever I'm using at the time helps her.

- CBD works alongside my other healthy habits and occasional supplements including EPA fish oils, macca powder, protein powder, creatine, ZMA tablets and multi vitamins.

- It doesn't make me hungry or suppress my appetite. I don't taste CBD in edibles. The CBD water that I tried didn't taste particularly nice. I'm not a big fan of bottled water though.

- CBD won't cure a hangover unfortunately. And pre-loading with CBD the night before doesn't lessen the chances of or make the ensuing hangover any easier. Milk Thistle is much better in this regard.

- It won't directly affect your sex drive one way or the other. If you take too much oil you might not be bothered doing anything at all apart from sleeping (intense exercise along with lots of seafood or magnesium, zinc and B6 supplements can help your libido)

- It can help me concentrate better and be more productive. It can help me focus during heavy exercise. It helps me with recovery from strength training and it can contribute to a feeling of wellness and positivity.

- Long term use has so far produced no side real effects or problems apart from it being quite expensive for my needs. If my stress levels become severe again, I'll continue to self-medicate as I have done already. I will try to avoid unnatural conventional medications.

- Different products and brands seem to vary slightly in taste and strengths despite showing the same percentage of CBD. Carrier oils used will affect the taste. Some oils darker in color e.g. rapeseed carrier oil is darker than coconut or olive oil. On top of this, people sometimes report that effects were different for them than what others claim. Again, it takes some experimentation to find the right brand that works for you and the sweet spot in the dosage.

- Lotions and salves do work but not as well as tinctures and capsules in my experience.

- CBD makes your skin, hair and nails look a bit healthier. It can generally increase your vitality and energy levels and help towards giving you a healthy glow.

- Oh, and CBD Hemp Oil will not make you high!

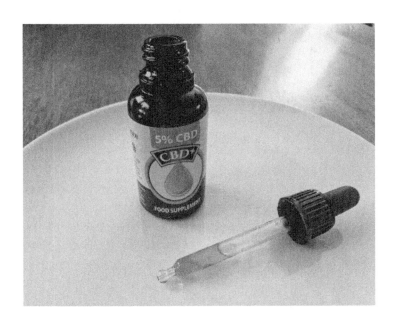

Phew! Now let's get back to Intermittent Fasting shall we?

Chapter 11:

Maintaining a Balanced Diet

Just because you are fasting, and possibly even on the ketogenic diet as well, doesn't mean you just eat salad. Salad is most certainly not a balanced diet. Lettuce may contain few calories but compared to other foods it is much lower in nutrition. It's also important to keep in mind that currently in America there is a common occurrence of lettuce becoming contaminated with salmonella and other bacteria.

While you may keep salad and lettuce within your diet, you need to be sure that you balance it out with plenty of other plant-based foods and proteins. We know that meat has many vital nutrients. We tend to only think of plant-based products and dairy when it comes to the nutritional contents of our diets, however meat provides many important nutrients we require.

We all know that meat contains a high amount of protein with all of the amino acids our bodies require. Beef contains an average of twenty-six percent protein. This means that for each one-hundred grams of beef there are twenty-six grams of essential amino acids which form the protein we so desperately require. An average three-ounce serving (eighty-five grams) contains twenty-two grams of protein. You will also find the healthy fats oleic acid, stearic acid, and palmitic acid to various degrees within beef depending on the fat level and whether it is a lean cut or not.

Yet, beef contains much more than the macronutrients of protein and fat; it also contains many micronutrients. These micronutrients are essential vitamins and minerals.

We tend to think of these as coming in plant-based food sources, such as vegetables or grains, but they are quite high in meats, as well. Not only that, but these essential nutrients are often better absorbed by our bodies when they originate from within meat rather than plant-based sources. Examples of micronutrients found in high quantities within beef include:

- **Vitamin B6:** This vitamin, like many B vitamins, is essential for human health. This type of B vitamin specifically participates in the formation of blood.
- **Vitamin B12:** We all know the importance of vitamin B12, but did you know it only occurs in animal-derived foods such as meat? This vitamin is imperative for both the formation of our blood and also the functioning of the nervous system and brain.
- **Iron:** While many people know we need iron, fewer know that there are two different types, heme and non-heme. You will find heme iron in meats and other animal-based products, whereas non-heme is found in plant-based ingredients. Heme, which is in large quantities in beef, is the most helpful type of iron since it is easily absorbed into the body. On the other hand, non-heme which is in kale, spinach, and other plant-based foods is not easily absorbed and often goes to waste by the body.
- **Zinc:** In order to stay healthy, fight off infections, and grow our bodies require zinc. You can find this essential nutrient in many immune system supporting supplements to help

fight off the flu and common cold. But your body can more easily absorb this mineral when you eat it naturally within food rather than in a supplement.

- **Selenium:** We may only require a small amount of selenium within our diets, but most foods don't contain the amount we need. Beef is an excellent source of this nutrient without having too much. This is important because selenium affects our metabolism, thyroid health, protects against disease, and more.

- **Niacin:** While this vitamin is commonly known as niacin, it is also one of the B vitamins, specifically vitamin B3. This nutrient is vital because every part of the human body requires it for survival. This vitamin helps to manage our cholesterol levels, manage heart health, increase brain health, and more. The best sources of niacin include beef, chicken, tuna, and salmon.

- **Glutathione:** Like plants, animal-based ingredients also contain important antioxidants which are used to fight disease. Glutathione is one of the most well-known and powerful antioxidants which is found in high number in meat, especially in grass-fed meat.

- **Creatine:** This antioxidant is vital for muscle health and energy. This nutrient also beneficially impacts out brain health, bone density, heart, mental health, lungs, and more. Bodybuilders often choose to eat large amounts of creatine or supplement with it, in order to get an extra boost for their muscles.

- **Taurine:** You may recognize taurine as being an ingredient common in energy drinks. It is a natural nutrient found within meat and fish which had many beneficial effects on the human body. This nutrient is especially helpful for heart health, blood health, and for people with certain chronic illnesses such as cystic fibrosis and congestive heart failure.

As you can see, there are many nutrients found within not only plant-based foods but meat as well. It's important not to forsake a balanced diet and only eat salad in order to lose weight. If you try to eat salad in order to cut down on your calories, you are likely to only create nutritional deficiencies and overly restrict your calorie consumption. Once calorie consumption is too highly restricted for a long period of time, your hormones will become unbalanced, and you will have difficulty losing weight. Instead, prioritize eating a balanced diet either following the ketogenic lifestyle or with the main healthy food groups of meat, eggs, grains, legumes, vegetables, fruits, and healthy fats.

You will naturally be time restricting your caloric intake while you are fasting, which will help you lose weight. When you are not fasting you shouldn't be restricting your calorie intake. Instead, focus on eating a balance of healthy whole foods in a moderate and appropriate amount.

Some people may develop malnutrition while practicing intermittent fasting or the ketogenic diet. This is not the fault of either the lifestyle or the person. The person who is following these principles simply does not have a full understanding of how to safely utilize them. They may choose to eat junk food when they are not fasting or eat salad with little else. This will naturally lead to deficiencies as they are not eating a wide variety of whole foods. Therefore, it is important to understand that when you are practicing this lifestyle, you must prioritize nutrition. Don't resort to packaged foods just because they label themselves as "natural," "organic," or "low-carb."

Be sure to eat an average of eight servings of fruits and vegetables a day, along with plenty of healthy meat, and grains and legumes if you are not following the ketogenic diet.

If you decide to pair the ketogenic diet with intermittent fasting, you may be reluctant to include many high-fat foods. But it is imperative to remember that fat and protein will be your two main fuel sources. Your body requires the calories and nutrition in order to not only thrive but to function at all. Prioritize getting healthy fats from meats, fish, eggs, nuts, seeds, fruits, vegetables, and healthy oils. These fats will enable your body to create more ketones, which will then keep you full and satisfied during long fasting periods.

For those pairing the ketogenic diet with intermittent fasting, remember to know your macro ratio and to track it. Later on, during the resources chapter at the end of the book, we will provide you with tools to both learn your macro ratio and to track it. This is imperative because otherwise, you can easily eat either too little or too much fat. The same is true of protein. You are unlikely to eat too much protein, but many people fail to eat enough which results in muscle loss and fatigue. Although, by simply tracking what you eat in accordance with your macro ratio you can ensure that during your eating windows between fasts that you are eating all of the nutrients your body requires.

If you find you are not losing weight, it may be because you have been lax in tracking your macros. This is the most common reason for a weight loss stall on the ketogenic diet. It may get old after a while to track what you are eating, but it is a quick, simple, and important process. By tracking your macros, you will be on the road toward success.

Dehydration and electrolyte imbalances are common for those who begin intermittent fasting or the ketogenic diet without a full understanding of what it does to the body. During the beginning of both of these processes, you will lose a large amount of water weight. This is weight is water molecules that have attached to glucose molecules within your body. But, when you are in a fasted or ketogenic state, your body will use up the glucose and, in the process, shed the water molecules. This weight adds up and can result in a person losing five to fifteen pounds within a week or two. It can be exciting to lose weight quickly, but remember that this is not weight from fat, but the water.
Therefore, since our bodies are losing quite a bit of hydration from losing water weight, it's important that we refuel. If you don't refuel on water you will become dehydrated, fatigued, develop headaches, constipation, kidney stones, bad breath, muscle cramps, and more.

Keep water on you at all times so that if you begin to feel the symptoms of dehydration, you can remedy the situation. If you are someone who dislikes plain water, there are other zero-calorie options that you can enjoy during your fast such as lemon water, unsweetened iced tea, Ultima Replenisher electrolyte drinks, Sweet Leaf stevia water drops, and Stur Water Enhancer.

Along with dehydration, you must be conscious of potential electrolyte imbalances. These are common when a person loses a lot of water weight because when you lose the water molecules, you also lose the electrolytes that were attached to them. If you increase your hydration without boosting your electrolyte intake, you will only be compounding upon the problem by causing a worsening of the imbalance. Thankfully, you can easily and simply increase your electrolyte intake as long as you have a little knowledge.

First, know that electrolytes are one of the most essential nutrient categories for the human body. These are minerals that are electrically charged within the water our bodies naturally contain. This allows the cells to communicate with one another and send nerve impulse transmissions. Without these electrolytes, our bodies would be completely unable to function, and our hearts would fail.

In order to keep a balance of electrolytes, it is important to consume sodium, magnesium, potassium, and calcium. You should easily be able to get calcium within your diet, so it is more important to focus on the remaining electrolytes.

You may be worried about sodium because you've heard that sodium causes heart problems, but the truth is that a lack of sodium causes an equal number of problems. Therefore, our goal should be to gain a balance of sodium. Thankfully, when you are practicing intermittent fasting with a healthy diet, you are unlikely to consume too much sodium. This is largely because junk food contains a much higher degree of sodium than whole foods, but also because your body won't be holding onto as much sodium.

When you are insulin resistant, your body tries to keep all of the sodium you consume, until you have too much built up within your body. As you treat your insulin resistance and lose weight your body will naturally begin to let go of the sodium. The recommended amount of sodium is between four and six grams a day, which is best to get from a healthy source. Try choosing a salt rich in minerals, such as pink Himalayan sea salt. However, you can always choose to use regular sea salt.

You will naturally find potassium within many healthy foods, not just bananas. You can easily consume your daily requirements with avocados, wild-caught salmon, mushrooms, dark leafy greens, sweet potatoes, eggplant, and more. The recommended daily serving is an average of four grams daily.

Lastly, you can easily find your daily requirement of magnesium within almonds, quinoa, whole wheat, black beans, avocados, and edamame. You should consume four-hundred milligrams daily.

It's important that you don't just integrate intermittent fasting into a junk food-filled life. Instead, try to maintain a balanced, healthy food diet or ketogenic diet while you practice intermittent fasting. This will not only help you to lose weight, but it will ensure that your meals are nutritionally balanced to prevent deficiencies and hunger.

Chapter 11:

Staying Positive and Motivated

Any life change is difficult. This is true whether you are moving, going to a new college, starting a new job, or beginning a new healthy lifestyle. But, while intermittent fasting may be quite a change from what you are used to, it can actually make life much easier. You will still be able to enjoy going out with friends to eat on occasion, but you also won't have to obsess over food and worry about eating every few hours. Instead, you can fully enjoy your meals during your feeding windows while being free to live your life free of worrying about food during your fasting period. I don't know about you, but I always feel annoyed when I am trying to get work done or run errands and have to stop and find something to eat. With intermittent fasting, you are allowed to have breaks to focus on your actual life and desires.

Within this chapter, you will find help in staying positive and how to stay motivated while you are making your lifestyle switch.

Don't Do Too Much Too Soon:
It can be a big change to begin intermittent fasting if you are someone used to eating on a regular basis. The human body adapts to our eating schedules, and over time it will begin to send us hunger signals at the times we usually eat, even if we don't require food yet. It's important to take things slowly and allow

your body to adapt naturally rather than jumping all into something that you are not yet ready for.

Instead of starting with a sixteen hour or twenty-four hour fast, begin with something shorter. You may simply start by skipping a meal on a day that you don't feel hungry. As an example, you may not feel like breakfast one day. Try skipping breakfast and only having a cup of tea or coffee until lunchtime. Or, you may start with a shorter twelve-hour fast. The shorter the fast, the fewer benefits you will experience, but you don't want to jump into a twenty-four hour fast just for the benefits. This will only discourage you. Remember, you can always work up to a twenty-four hour fast if that's what you want, but you don't have to accomplish it immediately.

If you begin a twelve hour fast immediately after dinner at seven-thirty in the evening, then you will be able to eat breakfast the following day at seven-thirty. This fast is rather short and easy to accomplish since you will be sleeping through most of it. Last on, if you want to increase the fast, you can slowly push back the time you eat every few days by thirty minutes until you reach a fourteen or sixteen-hour fast.

Be patient and don't push yourself too much too soon. Greater success and reward come to those who take it one step at a time.

Give Yourself Time:
Intermittent fasting is quite different than many people are used to, and it will take time to adjust. You may have a couple of difficult weeks while you adjust but give yourself the time you require. Throwing in the towel too soon will only lead you to feel

discouraged and prevent you from discovering the many amazing benefits that fasting has to offer. Instead, try to take up intermittent fasting when you have a couple of slow weeks. You don't want to begin when work or school is the busiest or during the holidays. Find a time when life is a little slow so that you can devote your time and energy to intermittent fasting. Allow yourself a full month to adjust, and before long you will be thankful that you didn't give up.

Don't Live by the Scale:

Some people may lose ten or fifteen pounds when they first begin intermittent fasting, while it may take other people more time. It's easy to be discouraged if you don't lose weight as quickly as others but remember that every person and everybody is different. The people who are losing weight more quickly upon beginning fasting are most likely losing water weight. You may not have as much water weight than them, but this is actually a good sign. If you have less water weight, your body is able to focus on actively burning fat. It may take longer to burn fat, but it offers much more of a reward.

Rather than living by the scale, try to only weigh yourself once or twice a week. Any more than this and you are likely to become obsessed with the number.

Keep in mind that the number on the scale is not necessarily accurate, as well. You may find that you have dropped a pant size, but the numbers remain the same. This is often caused by two factors.

Firstly, fasting can change your body composition to the better. You may find that you haven't necessarily lost fat, but that you have less fat around the dangerous area of your stomach. Secondly, muscle weighs more than fat. This means you may be losing fat, but if you are also gaining muscle the scale can either stay the same or even increase But, this is a good change.

Rather than relying on the numbers of the scale, try to use a tape measure to get all of your body measurements. This way you will know if your thighs, stomach, bust, hips, and other areas are becoming smaller, even if the scale doesn't show it.

You want to be able to see your progress as you achieve it. If you simply measure and weigh yourself without tracking it, the numbers will soon feel meaningless. Instead, use a little notebook where you can track these numbers toward your goals. If you like, you could even create a graph so you can see your numbers change at a glance.

Find a Buddy:

Making changes on your own is hard. If you are highly motivated and know your reasoning, you are certainly capable of making a diet change, with or without help. However, it will be a much easier and more positive experience if you can find a buddy to work together with during your time of transitioning to a healthier lifestyle. Whether you have a romantic partner, a friend, family member, or someone online as a partner, having a buddy can greatly improve the experience.

By having someone to work together with you can share recipes, discuss your experiences, encourage one another to keep going, and have someone who understands your lifestyle. If you are looking for someone like this and don't have anyone nearby, you can easily find other people who are experienced or new at intermittent fasting online. There are entire Facebook groups and social spheres online where you can meet people with the same goals and lifestyles. If you begin to participate in these groups and spheres, you will be able to reach out to a like-minded person and hopefully become a fasting buddy.

Although, if you are able to find someone who lives near you to become a buddy with, this is ideal. With a person like this, you can literally share meals, exercise together, and hang out together.

Practice Meditation:

Meditation has been used throughout the world for centuries to heal the mind, increase relaxation, to find balance during a time full of turmoil, and for increased health. Even before science proved the benefits of meditation and medicine provided further opportunities, people discovered the power this seemingly simple approach has to offer. Thousands of studies have shown that practicing meditation people can lower stress, improve sleep, increase results at work, boost weight loss, improve relationships, and increase focus.

You don't have to be religious to practice meditation, but if you are any religion can practice. There are multiple types of meditation, and you can find what works best for you. You don't even have to use a specific program. There are many meditation classes, online programs, and apps that you can choose to use. Or, you can learn meditation on your own and practice it by yourself, unassisted. Neither approach is superior, simply find which you are more comfortable with.

There are multiple ways in which meditation can improve your success at intermittent fasting, weight loss, and increased health. Three of their benefits include:

1: Increased Relief from Stress, Anxiety, and Depression

Many studies have found that regular meditation can help a person manage stress, anxiety, and depression. While if you are new to meditation, it may take you some time to see help with anxiety and depression, you should begin to see a lessening of stress right away. It's important to know that it takes time to learn to meditate in a way that helps you, but with practice, it is completely possible. Don't expect mystical results overnight, but you will likely see small benefits at the beginning that will only grow over time. One study reviewing forty-seven different mindfulness and meditation trials and over three and a half thousand participants found that people regularly experienced relief from anxiety and depression. These results were not only felt but could also be proven as effective due to a lessening in the stress hormone, cortisol.

2: Improved Sleep

Did you know that sleep is important for weight loss? If you don't sleep well your cortisol, ghrelin, and leptin hormones will become disrupted. When this occurs, your body will increase hunger signals, making it more difficult to fast. As if that weren't bad enough, it will also cause your body to hold onto weight making weight loss extremely difficult. Therefore, if you want you fasting and weight loss to be successful you must also focus on your sleep.

However, sleep may be difficult for some people. Insomnia is a common problem, especially in people who are making lifestyle changes. Thankfully, mindfulness and meditation have been shown to increase sleep and quality of sleep in many people. By practicing meditation before bedtime, you can calm the body and send it messages that it's time to sleep. Your breathing and mind will gradually calm down, and you will be able to sleep more soundly. This benefit may be slow at first, but as you get better at meditating, you will find that it's easier to utilize its benefits in order to increase sleep. A study by Harvard Medical School even found that focusing on a calming meditation phrase, such as "breathe in calm, breathe out tension" is much more effective than the old tradition of counting fluffy farm animals.

3: Increased Satisfaction and Well Being

Even when you are not actively meditation, by working meditation into your daily life studies have found that you are better able to regulate your emotions throughout the day. This can help you to have less stress, increase satisfaction, and lead a happier life. This will naturally make the process of beginning intermittent fasting easier and less overwhelming.

These are only a few benefits of mediation. If you hope to use this practice to increase your success, I recommend reading a book on the subject or downloading a guided meditation app or program.

Keep Busy:

Think about it, when you are lying in bed watching TV you are more likely to snack. Whereas, if you are running errands you are more likely to forget to eat. Rather than planning on beginning intermittent fasting while on vacation or have a slow weekend, plan it when you have activities going on. This doesn't mean you should begin fasting when you are overwhelmed at work, rather plan distractions. This could mean that you decide to work on your favorite hobby, video game, or go to some fun local attractions. Whatever you decide to do, having something to keep your mind occupied can help break the habit of eating when you don't truly need food.

Chapter 12:

Unconventional Ketogenic and Fasting Diets

If you are familiar with the ketogenic diet, you most likely have noticed that if often contains quite a number of meats, eggs, cheese, and heavy cream. This may be intimidating for people who have dairy allergies, are vegetarian, or vegan. While a keto vegan or dairy-free diet may look quite different, it is completely possible to attain if you put in the effort. It may take some time to figure out your individual lifestyle needs, but if you give it some time, you will find that some great protein-filled options can be included in a vegan ketogenic and fasting lifestyle. Within this chapter, we will discuss some of the best dairy-free and vegan protein sources along with some tips for attaining your new unconventional lifestyle.

If you only give it a try, you will soon find that it is entirely possible. But, be sure that you give it a real try. If you only attempt the new lifestyle for a week, you are unlikely to see its many benefits or learn how to fit it to your needs. Instead, attempt your new lifestyle for a month. This will give you all the time you need to figure out what exactly you require and how to make the diet fit into that. This time period will also give you ample time to experience the weight and health benefits that a fasting lifestyle paired with a vegan or dairy-free ketogenic diet has to offer.

One benefit of the dairy-free or vegan ketogenic diet is that many people on the ketogenic may experience weight loss stalls when they rely too heavily on dairy. These people often include cheese or heavy cream in nearly every meal. This, along with an excess of nuts, can easily cause weight loss stalls. But, with a dairy-free or vegan ketogenic diet, the temptation of eating too many of these ingredients is completely removed. Instead, you can focus on eating foods that will better benefit your weight loss and health. While meat and other animal-based products certainly have their own benefits, you are still able to attain the same benefits on a well-balanced plant-based lifestyle. This is especially helpful for people who struggle with allergies or chronic illnesses that prevent them from consuming certain animal products and for people who have a moral objection against animal-based products. Now, let's look into some of the best keto-friendly vegan protein options available.

Edamame

Edamame may be a bean, but they are much lower in net carbohydrates than most. This is because edamame is immature soybeans which are found still within their pod, containing a lot of fiber. While mature soybeans contain thirty-nine net carbohydrates, edamame only contains seven net carbs for an entire cup. This serving size also contains seventeen grams of protein, eight grams of fat, and many micronutrients. Some of the nutrients within edamame include magnesium, potassium, vitamin B6, zinc, iron, vitamin C, calcium, and vitamin K1. You can easily add edamame to a variety of dishes, not just stir-fry. But, better yet is that edamame has been shown to lower the risk of developing breast cancer, improve cholesterol, prevent bone loss, and manage the symptoms of menopause.

Tofu

Tofu is one of the most versatile low-carb protein options. You may not think you like tofu, but please give it a chance. In order to be enjoyable tofu needs to be prepared properly. Just because you didn't like tofu the first time, you tried it doesn't mean you will never like it. One of the many wonderful aspects of this ingredient is its ability to take on other flavors. This means that if you marinate tofu and top it with a sauce, you can enjoy a flavorful meal, no matter the cuisine. You can make anything from chocolate pudding to sesame "chicken" with tofu.

You can get many types of tofu, such as silken, firm, extra firm, fermented, smoked, and seasoned. One type of tofu cannot replace another, because they can all be used in different ways. For instance, extra firm tofu doesn't have the correct consistency to make pudding. On the other hand, silken tofu is too soft and won't hold up to be coated in sesame sauce and fried.

In general, a half-cup serving of tofu contains ten grams of protein and only two net carbs. The protein within tofu is extremely beneficial because usually, only animal-based products contain all nine of the amino acids the body requires. However, tofu is one of the few plant-based alternatives that contains these nine amino acids, as well. Along with these amino acids, tofu contains a decent amount of magnesium, zinc, calcium, iron, manganese, copper, phosphorous, and vitamin B1.

Along with lowering your risk of developing breast cancer, tofu can also improve brain health, treat kidney disease, increase weight loss, improve cardiovascular health, lower cholesterol, treat anemia, and more.

Tempeh

Most soy-based products originate from what is known as the Greater Chinese region. There are a couple of exceptions, one of which is tempeh. This vegan product was created in Indonesia by fermented soybeans. Tempeh if formed into a thick log while it is fermenting, which results in a more firm, chewy texture. This is ideal for people who desire a texture more like meat and don't care for the squishy feel of tofu. While tempeh does contain more carbs than tofu due to containing the whole soybean, it can be enjoyed in moderation on a vegan ketogenic diet.

The flavors of tempeh are different from tofu, due to it being fermented. However, when cooked with seasonings, marinated, or covered in a sauce you will not notice the fermentation flavor. Instead, it has a sweet, nutty flavor with a slight earthiness. The firm and chewy texture is a great meat substitute, even being ideal for vegan "bacon" If you are looking to cook tempeh, it is best when first marinated, but not necessary. Some people even choose to enjoy this ingredient straight out of the fridge and plain. But, if you would rather your tempeh cooked you can try pan-frying, grilling, roasting, frying, breading, or baking.

A single serving of tempeh (thirty ounces) contains six grams of fat, only three net carbs, and sixteen full grams of protein This is quite a good start, especially considering that it contains the full soybean. Like tofu, tempeh contains all nine essential amino acids, making it a wonderful option for vegans and people who choose to limit their meat consumption. This protein is also as easily absorbed as the protein found within meat products. By eating all nine amino acids within these foods, you will be able to maintain muscle health along with healthy cellular functioning.

Tempeh has been found to contain many nutrients and benefits. Part of the reason for this is that it has been fermented. By first fermenting the product it increases the ability of your body to easily absorb the nutrients. Not only that, but it contains many healthy probiotics that are good for your gut health. For this reason, tempeh can support regularity, prevent diarrhea, reduce bloating, treat irritable bowel syndrome, and even increase weight loss.

Mung Bean Sprouts

Mung bean sprouts are a wonderful low-carb and fresh option. You can add them to sandwiches, salads, stir-fries, use them in place of noodles, and more. This vegetable is used across East Asia. While it may be a little difficult to find in your local supermarket, you can easily make your own sprouts if you purchase mung beans online, at a health food store, or a local Asian marketplace. From there growing the bean sprouts is as easy as completing a childhood science project. I'm sure most of us remember growing bean sprouts in jars growing up.

While growing mung bean sprouts in a large batch might be slightly different, the basic principles remain the same. Although, it is important to know that occasionally mung bean sprouts may contain a type of bacteria when raw. Therefore, it is commonly recommended for the children, elderly, chronically ill, and pregnant people to only consume cooked mung bean sprouts. This fresh and crisp protein option contains three grams of protein and four net carbs per serving (one-hundred and four grams). While the carb to protein ratio isn't nearly as ideal as the previously mentioned protein options, it is still a helpful addition when enjoyed in moderation. Plus, mung bean sprouts are full of nutrients

Vegan Isolate Protein Powder

Isolated protein powders are much lower in carbs than others because they are a more purified form of protein. If you are looking for a protein powder be sure that it is not only vegan but also on isolate. One wonderful option is Hammer Nutrition's Vanilla Soy Protein Powder. This protein powder is originally made from soybean, but the carbohydrate portion has been removed so that it is the purified protein from the bean. Yet, despite being a more purified form, the manufacturers were able to keep the nutritional elements intact. This means that this protein powder still contains a high number of phytonutrients, iron, and other vitamins and minerals. It's also important to keep in mind that soybean-sourced protein contains all nine of the essential amino acids the body requires. Because of this, it is easy to add a couple of scoops of this protein powder to your day to increase your protein intake. A single scoop of this specific protein powder contains twenty-three grams of protein yet only two net carbs.

As you can see, going vegan on a fasting and ketogenic lifestyle may be different from what you are used to, but it is entirely possible and feasible. There is no reason to fear or hold back, you can achieve your dreams.

Chapter 13:

Ketogenic Recipes Ideal for Fasting

Whether you are solely enjoying intermittent fasting on its own or choose to pair it with the ketogenic diet, within this chapter, you will find all the recipes you need to capture both your heart and your taste buds. Eating healthfully and losing weight doesn't mean you need to sacrifice flavor. Trust me you should try these!

Easy Italian Omelet

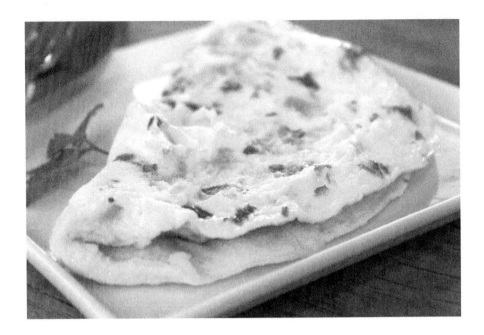

Who doesn't enjoy a luxurious omelet from time to time? Let me tell you, a decadent and flavorful omelet doesn't have to be difficult or time-consuming. With this rich Italian omelet, you can enjoy a host of flavors with minimal effort and time. This omelet is the perfect choice whether you wish to enjoy it for a weekend brunch with friends or by yourself on a Monday prior to beginning the workday.

Servings: 2 - Calories: 340 - Fat: 29 – Total Carbs: 4 - Net Carbs: 3 - Protein: 15

The Omelet Ingredients:
Mushrooms, sliced – 1 cup
Zucchini, sliced – 1 cup

Eggs, whole – 4, large

Grass-fed butter – 3 tablespoons

Water – 3 tablespoons

Sea salt - .25 teaspoons

Mozzarella, whole fat, shredded - .5 cup

Pepper, ground - .25 teaspoons

The Sauce Ingredients:

Tomato, chopped – 1, medium

Grass-fed butter – 1 tablespoon

Garlic, minced – 2 cloves

Fresh parsley, minced – 2 tablespoons

Basil, dried - .5 teaspoons

Sea salt - .25 teaspoon

The Instructions:

1. Place the sliced mushrooms and zucchini squash, along with two tablespoons of butter, in a large non-stick skillet and allow them to sauté until they become softened. Remove the vegetables from the skillet.

2. Melt the remaining tablespoon of butter in the skillet that you removed the vegetables from. Whisk together the eggs with the sea salt, water, and black pepper before pouring them into the skillet with the butter over medium-high heat. You will notice the edges of the eggs begin to set from the heat immediately.

3. As the eggs cook, you should use a spatula to slowly move them around so that they stay mostly flat, but to allow the entire portion of eggs to become evenly cooked. As the egg begins to completely set leave it alone so that you don't end up with holes.

4. Once the eggs set place the vegetables on one side and top it with the cheese. Using your spatula gently flip the other half of the omelet over the top of the cheese and vegetables and remove it from the heat.

5. After you remove the omelet from the skillet quickly combine the sauce ingredients of tomato, butter, sea salt, garlic, parsley, and basil. Allow them to cook together until heated through, about three to five minutes. Pour the sauce over the omelet and enjoy

Orange Cranberry Muffins

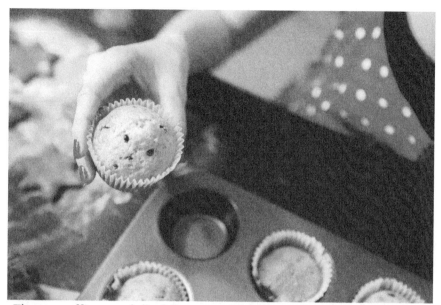

These muffins are full of flavor and bright, perfect for either summer or autumn with the zesty fresh orange and the tart cranberries. Not only that, but they are completely gluten and grain free

Servings: 6 – Calories: 183 – Fat: 14 – Total Carbs: 8 – Net Carbs: 4 – Protein: 5

The Ingredients:

Almond flour – .66 cup
Coconut flour – 3 tablespoons
Psyllium husk – 1 tablespoon
Baking powder - .5 teaspoon
Baking soda - .5 teaspoon
Sea salt - .25 teaspoon
Xanthan gum - .5 teaspoon

Pure sugar-free sweetener – .33 cup

Eggs, divided – 2, large

Apple cider vinegar – 1 teaspoon

Orange zest – 2 teaspoons

Vanilla extract – 1 teaspoon

Orange juice – 2 tablespoons

Water – 2 tablespoons

Grass-fed butter, melted – .25 cup

Fresh cranberries – .75 cup

The Instructions:

1. While you mix up, the orange cranberry muffins preheat the oven to three hundred- and fifty-degrees Fahrenheit and prepare a muffin tin with six cups with paper liners or by greasing it with butter and coating it with coconut flour.
2. After separating the eggs beat the egg whites in a very clean bowl until soft peaks are created and then set the bowl of whites aside.
3. In another medium-sized bowl combine the coconut flour, almond flour, baking powder, psyllium husk, xanthan gum, baking soda, and sea salt. Set this bowl of dry ingredients aside.
4. In another bowl use an electric mixer to beat together the Pure sugar-free sweetener and the egg yolks until they become pale and fluffy which should take about one to three minutes.
5. Into the egg yolk and Pure sweetener, bowl add in the vanilla extract, orange zest, apple cider vinegar, and melted butter. Slowly bold in the almond flour along with the water and orange juice.

6. Gently fold the egg whites into the mixture of egg yolks, flour, and liquid. It will be thick, but it will slowly loosen up as you fold in the egg whites. After the egg whites are folded in gently fold in the fresh cranberries.
7. Spoon the cranberry orange batter between the six muffin cups and bake until it is set and cooked all the way through, about eighteen to twenty minutes. You can test the cranberry muffins by inserting a toothpick into the center and removing it; if the toothpick is removed clean, then the muffins are done cooking.

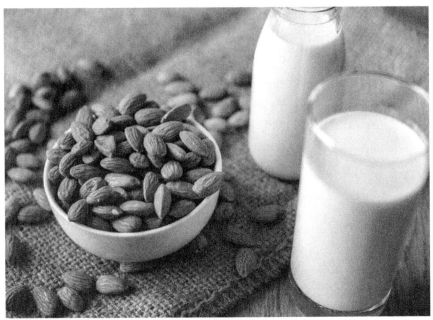

Easy Almond Flour Bread

Just because you are unable to eat grain on the ketogenic diet doesn't mean you can't have bread. This delicious bread is made with almond flour, making it low-carb and full of nutrients. Not only that, but this bread is incredibly easy and quick to mix up

Servings: 6 – Calories: 232 – Fat: 17 – Total Carbs: 13 – Net Carbs: 4 – Protein: 9

The Ingredients:

Eggs, divided – 2

Egg whites – 2

Baking powder - .5 teaspoon

Psyllium husk – 4 tablespoons

Xanthan gum - .5 teaspoon

Almond flour – 2 cups

Sea salt - .25 teaspoon
Warm water - .5 cup and 2 tablespoons

The Instructions:

1. While you mix up your almond flour bread preheat the oven to three hundred- and fifty-degrees Fahrenheit and prepare a small seven-inch by three-inch loaf pan with parchment paper. You can also use a regular nine-inch by five-inch loaf pan, although the bread will be a little flatter.
2. Beat the eggs until the egg white is fully combined into the egg yolk, and then add in the psyllium husk, almond flour, xanthan gum, baking powder, sea salt, and water. Only combine until the dough is smooth, not over-mixing it.
3. Scrape the batter into the prepared and parchment-lined baking sheet and bake it until a knife inserted into the center is removed clean, about forty-five minutes. However, you should keep an eye on the bread, and if it is already beginning to darken too much after thirty-five minutes, you can cover it with aluminum foil.
4. Allow the bread loaf to cool before slicing.

Smoked Salmon and Goat Cheese Appetizer

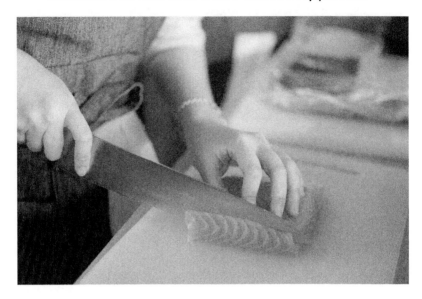

This delicious smoked salmon appetizer is luxurious, yet only takes a couple of minutes to prepare. As if that weren't a good enough reason to enjoy this appetizer, it is free of carbs and contains vital omega-3 fatty acids. Just because something is delicious doesn't mean it can't also be nutritious.

Servings: 6 – Calories: 107 – Fat: 6 – Total Carbs: 0 – Net Carbs: 0 – Protein: 11

The Ingredients:

Smoked salmon, thinly sliced into twelve pieces – 6 ounces
Goat cheese – 4 ounces
Lime juice – 1 tablespoon
Salmon caviar - .5 ounce
Chives, chopped – 12
Cayenne pepper - .5 teaspoon (optional)

The Instructions:

8. In a small bowl, combine four ounces of goat cheese, lime juice, and optional cayenne pepper until it is smooth and creamy.

9. Inside each of the twelve thinly sliced pieces of smoked salmon place a small scoop of the creamy goat cheese mixture. Roll each piece into an individual log.

10. Top the salmon goat cheese rolls with chopped chives and the salmon caviar. Store in the fridge up to two hours before serving.

Easy Kale Chips

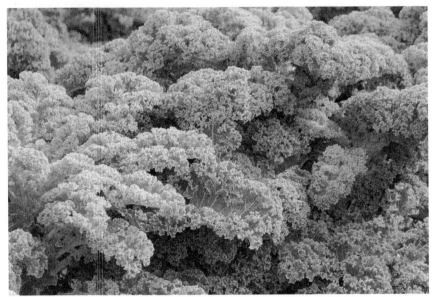

These delicious chips are perfect next to a sandwich or on their own when you are looking for a salty and crispy snack. While these make use of nutritional yeast for flavor, you can also try using your favorite spices such as curry powder or paprika.

Servings: 4 – Calories: 48 – Fat: 5 – Total Carbs: 3 – Net Carbs: 2 – Protein: 1

The Ingredients:

Large bunch of curly kale – 1 (about 6 ounces)
Avocado oil – 1.5 tablespoons
Sea salt – large pinch
Nutritional yeast – 1 tablespoon

The Instructions:

1. Preheat the oven to two-hundred- and twenty-five-degrees Fahrenheit while you mix up your kale chips.

2. After you completely wash and dry the kale tear it into small bite-sized pieces discarding the stems from the leaves.
3. Place the torn kale chips into a large bowl and toss them with the avocado oil, sea salt, and nutritional yeast until the seasoning is evenly coating the leaves.
4. Spread the seasoned kale over one or two baking sheets so that it is in a single layer and can become crispy. You don't want the kale leaves touching each other more than absolutely necessary. Otherwise it won't become crispy.
5. Bake the kale chips for fifteen minutes before tossing the kale leaves and allowing them to bake for an additional five to ten minutes until the leaves become golden-brown and crispy. You have to keep a close eye on them. Otherwise they can easily burn.
6. Remove the kale chips from the oven and let them slightly cool, which will allow them to become even more crispy. The chips are best enjoyed when they are fresh, although you can store them at room temperature for two to three days.

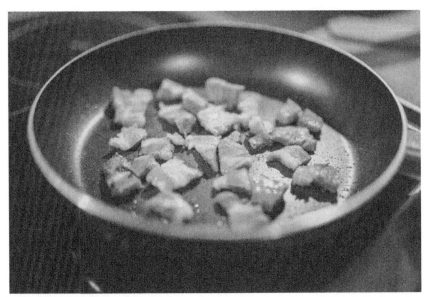

Feta Bacon Bites

Keto cheese dough is a magical low-carb dough perfect for savory and sweet treats alike. The dough cooks almost exactly like a buttery wheat dough, but it is completely grain-free and versatile in this recipe, the keto cheese dough is combined with bacon, feta cheese, and sriracha mayonnaise to create a rich and decadent appetizer.

Servings: 24 – Calories: 76 – Fat: 6 – Total Carbs: 1 – Net Carbs: 1 – Protein: 4

The Ingredients:

Mozzarella cheese, shredded – 2 cups

Almond flour - .75 cup

Feta cheese, crumbled - .25 cup

Bacon cooked and crumbled – 8 slices

Green onions, chopped - .25 cup

Black pepper and sea salt – to taste

Sriracha mayonnaise – 3 tablespoons

The Instructions:

1. While you assemble your feta bacon bites preheat a large oven to three-hundred- and fifty-degrees Fahrenheit.
2. Place the mozzarella cheese and almond flour in a non-stick skillet over medium heat and allow it to cook together until it turns into a form dough, about five minutes.
3. Remove the cheese dough from the heat, place it between two sheets of parchment paper, and roll it flat with a cooling rack until it's about ¼ of an inch thick.
4. Using a small round cookie cutter slice the dough into twenty-four circles. If you end up with extra dough, you can warm it back up, roll it out again, and then slice out the remaining circles of dough.
5. Place the circles of dough into a mini muffin tin so that it creates mini crusts. Although, you could also lay the circles out flat on a baking sheet.
6. Top the dough with the crumbled feta, crumbled bacon, chopped green onions, and spices. Bake the appetizers in the oven until the edges are lightly browned, about fifteen minutes. Serve the Feta Bacon Bites with sriracha mayonnaise.

Chili Cheese Muffins

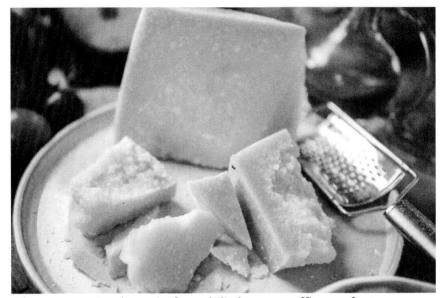

These are a simple grain-free chili cheese muffin, perfect to go alongside a bowl of low-carb chili, a pot of soup, or with some eggs for breakfast. Plus, with only six ingredients they are easy and quick to whip up

Servings: 9 – Calories: 203 – Fat: 16 – Total Carbs: 3 – Net Carbs: 2 – Protein: 11

The Ingredients:

Almond flour – 1.25 cup

Eggs – 3, large

Baking soda - .5 teaspoon

Sea salt - .5 teaspoon

Cheddar cheese, grated – 2 cups (8 ounces)

Red pepper flakes – 2 tablespoons

The Instructions:

1. Combine the almond flour, sea salt, and baking soda in a bowl while the oven preheats at three-hundred- and fifty-degrees Fahrenheit.
2. Add the eggs, shredded cheddar cheese, and red pepper flakes into the bowl and combine completely.
3. Divide the muffin batter between nine lined muffin cups and bake until cooked all the way through and a toothpick once inserted is removed clean. This cooking process should take approximately twenty-five to thirty minutes.

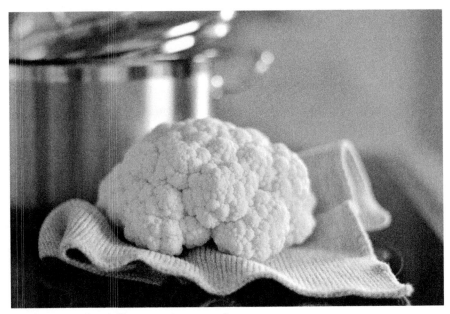

Cheesy Cauliflower Casserole

If you are someone who loves potatoes, you will have to try this cauliflower casserole which will win over practically any potato lover. If you are making it for your family, you don't even have to tell them that you used cauliflower rather than potatoes

Servings: 6 – Calories: 236 – Fat: 19 – Total Carbs: 7 – Net Carbs: 5 – Protein: 10

The Ingredients:

Cauliflower – 1 head

Cheddar cheese, shredded -1 cup

Cream cheese – 4 ounces

Parmesan cheese, grated - .25 cup

Sour cream - .5 cup

Heavy cream – 1 tablespoon

Bacon, cooked and chopped – 6 slices

Green onions, chopped - .25 cup

Garlic, minced – 3 cloves

Sea salt – to taste

The Instructions:

1. Preheat the oven to three hundred- and fifty-degrees Fahrenheit while you prepare the cauliflower and set aside an eight-inch square casserole dish.

2. Remove the stem from the cauliflower, cut it into florets, and boil it in salted water until it becomes tender which should take fifteen to twenty minutes.

3. In a large metal or glass bowl mash the cauliflower and add in the cream cheese, grated Parmesan cheese, sour cream, heavy cream, ¾ of the bacon, garlic, and green onions. Spread the mixture into the prepared casserole dish.

4. Top the cauliflower casserole dish with the remaining bacon and the shredded cheddar cheese and allow it to bake until the cheese is bubbly and golden about fifteen to twenty minutes.

Conclusion

Congratulations on finishing *Intermittent Fasting for Beginners*, I hope that you have found all the answers that you were seeking and that you are inspired you to act now and enjoy the benefits of this amazing eating method. If you enjoyed this book, please consider leaving it a review.

Intermittent fasting may be a different lifestyle than you are accustomed to, especially if you pair it with the ketogenic diet or a vegan lifestyle. But that doesn't mean it is impossible or even has to be difficult. Yes, any lifestyle change is difficult to begin however, in the long-run intermittent fasting will become easier and it will simplifiy your life. You will find that the longer you practice fasting, the easier it will become, the more benefits you will see, and the more you will believe in your new lifestyle.

There is no reason to go on crash diets which will only damage your metabolism and health over time. Intermittent fasting has been found to be safe and healthy time and again. Rather than damaging your health you can take steps to improve your life long into the future. You don't have to go on a crash diet that will only make you gain more weight soon after finishing. Intermittent fasting is maintainable and offers long-term results.

What are you waiting for? A new world of health, weight loss, and stress-free living is waiting for you. All you have to do now is to take action with the tools you have learned in this book.

Again, thank you for taking the time to read *Intermittent Fasting for Beginners*

Thank you for taking the time to read this book. If you have enjoyed the read, then please nip on to amazon here http://www.Amazon.com/gp/customer-reviews/write-a-review.html?asin=B07NQQY5TZ

Thank you and I wish you the very best of luck!

Here's a final thought for you before you leave:

You can be the person you deserve to be.
You have the power to change your life.
You don't need to settle for anything less.
Why wait? Start right now!

Robert McGowan

Did you like this book? You might like other published works from the author.

Have you ever dreamed of owning a Porsche but thought they were too expensive to buy and run? I'll show you how a Porsche can be free motoring based on my own experience. Discover how to find and buy the right Porsche and get your money back come resale. Learn how to spot the telltale signs of IMS and bore scoring and which cars have the best investment potential.

US link http://www.amazon.com/dp/1980940517

UK link http://www.amazon.co.uk/dp/1980940517

Have you heard about Cryptocurrency or Bitcoin or Blockchain Technology, but you are still vague about what they are and how they work?

Then this book is for you!

US link http://www.amazon.com/dp/1983247804
UK link http://www.amazon.co.uk/dp/1983247804

Discover exactly how to buy and use CBD Hemp oil to treat anxiety, depression, insomnia and more. Learn from an experienced hemp oil user and practicing Herbalist and Nutritionist.

Ebook is FREE with the paperback

UK link http://www.amazon.co.uk/dp/1729365809
US link http://www.amazon.com/dp/1729365809

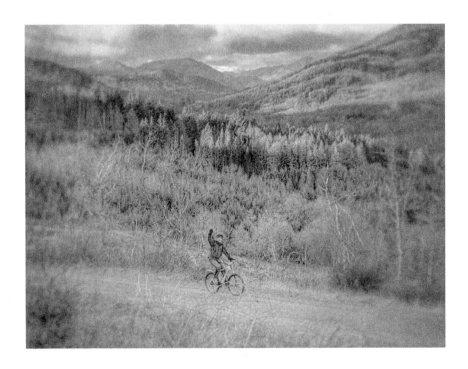

Common Terms

The Macro Ratio:
The three main nutrients, carbohydrates, protein, and fats.

Micronutrients:
The vital vitamins, minerals, antioxidants, and phytonutrients that your body requires.

Net Carbs:
The number of carbs after fiber has been removed from the equation. This means if an ingredient has ten total carbs, but six grams of fiber the net carb count will only be four.

Fasting Window:
The time in which you eat nothing or drink nothing with calories. Fasting windows last for different time periods, commonly between twelve and twenty-four hours.

Feeding Window:
The time between fasts when you eat your nutritionally balanced meals.

IF:
IF stands for Intermittent Fasting.

Ketones:
A fuel source that your liver produces with fat cells to provide fuel for cells which cannot use fat alone.

Ketosis:

The process of when you no longer have glucose within your cells, so your liver begins to make ketones for fuel instead.

Keto-Adapted:

The state you are in after you have been on the ketogenic diet for a few weeks and your body has fully adjusted to using ketones for fuel rather than glucose.

Further Resources

Perfect Keto Calculator: https://perfectketo.com/keto-macro-calculator/

Ruled.Me Keto Calculator: https://www.ruled.me/keto-calculator/

The Health Benefits of Meditation: https://mindworks.org/blog/health-benefits-of-meditation/

The Truth About Protein Absorption: https://www.muscleforlife.com/the-truth-about-protein-absorption-how-often-you-should-eat-protein-to-build-muscle/

Intermittent Fasting for People with Type II Diabetes: https://casereports.bmj.com/content/2018/bcr-2017-221854.full

How Fasting Can Fight Cancer: https://news.usc.edu/103972/fasting-like-diet-turns-the-immune-system-against-cancer/

Fasting and Cancer Treatment: https://www.ncbi.nlm.nih.gov/pmc/articles/PMC2815756/

Fasting for PCOS: https://www.researchgate.net/publication/317858823_Fasting_as_possible_complementary_approach_for_polycystic_ovary_syndrome_Hope_or_hype

Fasting for Better Gut Bacteria and MS Treatment: https://www.nationalmssociety.org/About-the-Society/News/Intermittent-Fasting-Changes-Gut-Bacteria-and-Redu

Fasting for Fatty Liver Disease: https://www.sciencedaily.com/releases/2016/05/160509085347.htm

Fasting for Mood Disorders:
https://www.sciencedirect.com/science/article/pii/S016517
8112008153
Skipping Breakfast to Relieve Depression:
https://psychcentral.com/lib/could-skipping-breakfast-relieve-depression/

Intermittent Fasting Induces Neuronal Autophagy:
https://www.ncbi.nlm.nih.gov/pmc/articles/PMC3106288/

Fasting Reduces Inflammation and Oxidative Stress:
https://www.ncbi.nlm.nih.gov/pubmed/17291990/

Fasting Reduces Risk of Cardiovascular Disease and Lowers
Inflammation: https://www.ncbi.nlm.nih.gov/pubmed/17374948

Intermittent Fasting is Effective for Weight Loss:
https://www.ncbi.nlm.nih.gov/pubmed/19793855

Fasting and Cancer Treatment:
https://www.ncbi.nlm.nih.gov/pubmed/20157582/

Intermittent Fasting Protects Rats Against Alzheimer's Disease:
https://www.ncbi.nlm.nih.gov/pubmed/17306982

Exercising while Fasted has Increased Benefits:
https://leangains.com/fasted-training-for-superior-insulin-sensitivity-and-nutrient-partitioning/

Regular Fasting is Good for Your Health and Heart:
https://www.sciencedaily.com/releases/2011/04/110403090259.htm